PRAISES for *WOUNDED WORKERS*

Wounded Workers is a wise, entertaining memoir that teaches while it describes Dr. Larsen's journey at becoming an occupational psychiatrist. From "slap therapy" to "post traumatic growth", it introduces new ideas that challenge our field. The clinical tales are often gripping and self-revelatory. This is a wonderful read for clinicians, trainees and anyone interested in the richness that is the practice of psychiatry today.

Steven S. Sharfstein, M.D.
President Emeritus, Sheppard Pratt Health System
Past President, American Psychiatric Association
Past President, American College of Psychiatrists

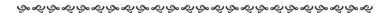

Wounded Workers is an entertaining and insightful deep dive into the world of workers hurt at work and the psychic difficulties they face. Dr. Larsen writes with experience as a forensic psychiatrist at the intersection of medicine and law, and his stories about the workers, written with wit and compassion, make the book sparkle.

Julius Young, Esq.
Boxer & Gerson

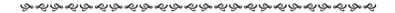

Although the current COVID-19 pandemic has increased appreciation of first responders, similar to what was seen post 9-11, Dr. Larsen has dedicated this book, and much of his professional career, to American workers and their collective ongoing contribution to our greater good. We can honor them through a thoughtful read of the cases he shares, reminding ourselves to not take what they do for all of us for granted.

David Baron, D.O.
Provost – Western University of Health Sciences
Emeritus Professor of Psychiatry, University of Southern California.

In *Wounded Workers* Dr. Bob Larsen is engaging, entertaining, compassionate and generous about his own journey, as well as about people whom he evaluated and treated. He is a psychiatrist with heart and brains. I spent 34 years representing injured workers in San Francisco, and I can tell you that every vignette Dr. Bob relates is representative and true. This well-written book is must reading for anyone interested in the price paid daily by many working men and women in America for doing their job. Well done, Dr. Bob!

Yale Jones, Esq.
Retired labor law attorney and senior partner, Jones, Clifford, LLP

ఄ⇌ఄ⇌ఄ⇌ఄ⇌ఄ⇌ఄ⇌ఄ⇌ఄ⇌ఄ⇌ఄ⇌ఄ⇌ఄ⇌ఄ

One will finish this excellent book not only being touched by the compassion and humanity of this dedicated psychiatrist but also being grateful for seeing how necessary psychiatry often is for individuals who have been physically injured.

Gary E. Wise, Ph.D, Professor & Head, Emeritus,
School of Veterinary Medicine, Louisiana State University

WOUNDED WORKERS

I hope these tales speak to you.

Dr. Bob

WOUNDED WORKERS
Tales from a Working Man's Shrink

Dr. Bob Larsen

Working Man's Press

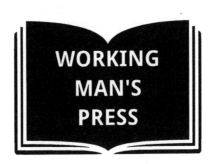

WORKING
MAN'S
PRESS

WOUNDED WORKERS
Tales from a Working Man's Shrink

Published 2021 by Robert C. Larsen
Working Man's Press
P.O. Box 31193
Santa Fe, NM 87594
https://workingmansshrink.com
https://www.facebook.com/workingmansshrink

Library of Congress Control Number: 2020908795

ISBN-13: 978-1-7348175-0-8 (Paperback Book)
978-1-7348175-1-5 (eBook/Kindle)
978-1-7348175-2-2 (eBook/ePub)
978-1-7348175-3-9 (Hardback Book)

Disclaimer:

This book is not designed to and does not provide medical advice, diagnostic assessment, treatment or other clinical services. *Wounded Workers*, its website linkages, the author Robert C. Larsen, and the publisher Working Man's Press provide information for reading and educational purposes only. The information provided is not a substitute for medical or psychiatric care, and you should not use it in place of consultation or advice from your physician or health care providers. Dr. Larsen and Working Man's Press are not responsible for any clinical advice, diagnosis, treatment, products, or services you obtained by reading this book. Neither the Food and Drug Administration nor any other government agency has evaluated statements made in this book.

DEDICATION

This book is dedicated to all workers who produce goods, provide services, and administer systems in America while risking their lives, physical health, and emotional well-being.

FOREWORD

I love books that, besides being well-written and entertaining, help me learn something important. *Wounded Workers* is one of those! Dr. Bob Larsen skillfully interweaves the inspiring story of his development from a self-described nerdy kid to a well-regarded psychiatrist and advocate for working people. The text explodes with fascinating stories of clients Dr. Bob has helped and with tales of those who mentored and helped him.

A crusader for making mental health care accessible as a basic human right, Dr. Bob's advocacy sought to persuade insurance companies and employers to consider the long-term psychological impact of debilitating work-related injuries.

Some of the many moving encounters highlight the amazing resilience of maimed and traumatized workers who, instead of giving up, found value in the life that was left for them. Dr. Bob's descriptions of how his clients struggled to deal with the psychological effects of loss of limbs, scarring accidents, and other traumatic events testify to the need for major and compassionate change. Many of the stories focus on "essential workers," people who need the practical and kind advice of a working man's shrink more than ever. His astute observations on overcoming victimization and the inspiring reality of Post Traumatic Growth resonated deeply with me, especially in the trying times of COVID grief and isolation.

Wounded Workers will resonate with general readers as well as anyone with a special interest in mental health care and making it more accessible as a basic human right.

Anne Hillerman
N. Y. Times Best-Selling Author

INTRODUCTION

Wounded Workers is a compilation of true stories — of bank tellers, police officers, firefighters, managers, farm workers, and many others — that chronicles how we Americans handle extreme misfortune while simply trying to do our jobs. The book includes accounts of employees involved in robberies, motor vehicle accidents, machinery malfunctions, and other life-changing adverse events. As you read, you will no doubt feel a range of emotions, as the tales range from heartbreaking to inspirational.

Over my long career as a physician and psychiatrist, I have been blessed to be of service to working people subjected to physical injury, severe psychological stress, cumulative exposure to interpersonal conflict, and other challenges. The cases portrayed in the chapters that follow are representative of workers who demand attention and understanding.

Most of the individuals portrayed in *Wounded Workers* were referred to my office through legal and administrative channels. The cases often involved claims of injury, typically physical, mental, or both. The California workers' compensation system classifies doctors as either treating or evaluating clinicians on a given case. In the chapter titled That's Where the Money Is, I was the psychiatrist who treated the bank teller robbed multiple times. In the chapter Of Course It's Personal, involving a firefighter and paramedic who sought help related to the death of a family member, I was the treating doctor. In a number of other chapters, such as I Am Unlovable and Raped with a Gun, the cases are described from my perspective as the evaluating psychiatrist.

The workers' compensation system, developed decades ago, is generally regarded as a "great compromise" between management and labor. Injured workers receive expeditious medical care and disability benefits in exchange for relinquishing their rights to sue employers in Superior Court. But as you will see, the system does not always work as intended. Even when it does, multiple players are involved, including the treating doctors, other clinicians, insurance company representatives, attorneys for both the employer and the injured worker, utilization review personnel, and an administrative law judge. Complex cases might be highly litigated and require review by the Workers' Compensation Appeals Board for the State of California.

There is no such thing as a simple psychiatric claim. Whether administered as a workers' comp claim or one that is adjudicated through other civil proceedings, most claims of psychological injury are initially denied, in whole or in part. My role in most of these sagas was to comb through voluminous records, meet with the claimant, and then issue a report that typically arrived at a diagnosis while answering the central question of who was responsible. The cases were referred by applicant attorneys representing the employee, defense attorneys for the employer and insurer, or by a judge. The California system allows the parties to select an Agreed Medical Examiner (AME) of a given medical specialty to offer opinions on the medical/legal issues of diagnosis, causation of injury, temporary disability, treatment, permanent disability, and fitness for duty. After years of practice, I found myself designated as an AME in most of my forensic work-related cases. Yet sometimes, it seemed I pleased no one.

Where legal matters are prominent, there is always the potential for bias on the part of doctors involved. Treating doctors might recommend more-extensive care than necessary. Evaluating doctors might wish to please a referral source. Doctors are human and can be vulnerable to prejudice for or against a particular employee. Sometimes, doctors are not aware of how counter-transference might affect our opinions. By the way, the use of clinical jargon such as "counter-transference" (unconscious feelings about a patient based upon what he/she represents to the doctor) is minimized in this book. You won't have to take an introductory class on mental health law on-line or at the local community college to appreciate what follows.

I come from working-class roots, and my own story is intertwined with those of the patients referred for treatment and the claimants seen for evaluation. My mother was an immigrant from Italy who never attended high school and was 14 when she found a job in a factory. My father enlisted in the U.S. Army as a teenager and was a soldier for the duration of World War II. Growing up in the Chicago area during the 1950s and 1960s, I was expected to show respect for adults who worked in manufacturing plants, offices, farm settings, and at construction sites. The COVID-19 pandemic has brought increased attention to and appreciation for first responders and employees in hospitals, research labs, grocery stores, delivery jobs, and many other relied-upon industries. This book is an expression of my continued respect for American workers, and a recognition of their contributions to our greater good.

I hope you enjoy the stories that follow, and in some cases you might put yourself in the shoes of the men and women I have worked with – and perhaps you can feel their frustration, pain, sorrow, and even their joy and victories.

LIST OF PHOTOGRAPHS

The photographs in *Wounded Workers* introduce each chapter through an image that:

- Is representative of the chapter title,
- Conveys a story or theme from the chapter,
- And/or Is an abstract expression of an emotion portrayed in, or experienced by reading, the chapter.

The following list details the subject of photographic images by chapter.

Photographs in this book were made by Dr. Bob Larsen, except for the images for Chapters 2 & 30, which were captured by Kim Larsen.

Contents

PRIVACY STATEMENT

Great care was taken to protect the employees described in *Wounded Workers*. Most names were changed. In certain cases, employers' names were altered. Most of the encounters and incidents took place in a time frame not specified. All modifications were done to preserve confidentiality.

On the other hand, essential aspects of each case were preserved, including the nature of the injurious event, the medical treatment rendered, approximate age of the worker, and job title. Gender was not altered.

In summary, I made a sincere effort to preserve the privacy of those whose stories I tell here. Please keep in mind I wrote accurate depictions of tales told by people doing their jobs and who, through no fault of their own, fell upon misfortune. There was no basis for blame or shame.

Dr. Bob Larsen

"In the end, we are not defined by the particular product or service we create, but rather the manner in which we affect those we serve. If you are engaging in meaningful work, those for whom you provide service will define your value."

— *Dr. Bob Larsen*

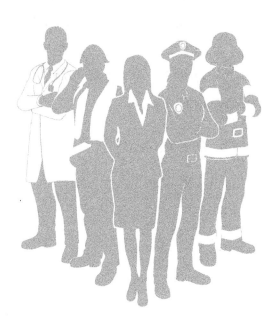

1 | Because That's Where the Money Is

Mariana came into my office scared, tense, and understandably mistrustful. This wasn't the first time she'd been involved in an armed robbery. It was the fourth time in a decade. Just her luck. And the last person to rob her was someone she least expected. As Willie Sutton was claimed to have replied when asked by a reporter why he robbed banks, "Because that's where the money is." Banks get held up. According to FBI statistics, in the decade ending in 2018, 3,000 to more than 6,000 banks, savings and loans, and credit unions are robbed each year across America. In Mariana's case, the insurer for Crocker Bank in San Francisco referred her to me. She was accompanied by George, her male partner, when she visited my office in an old Victorian off Fillmore Street in the Pacific Heights District. We met there every week or two for the next two years.

Mariana was on duty in April 1974 when members of the Symbionese Liberation Army (SLA) conducted a takeover-style robbery of the downtown branch of Hibernia Bank. During our consultation, she told me she felt grateful to be alive after the angry masked thieves had left without shooting anyone. "Maybe our training got us through," she told me. The incident captured by surveillance cameras was played out in newspapers and on television. A kidnapped newspaper heiress was shown among members of the SLA, actively participating in the robbery, which was a federal crime.

Mariana told me that as a young girl in China many years earlier in WW II, she had seen hostile Japanese soldiers. Those soldiers weren't wearing ski masks, like the bank robbers were, but they made clear who was in charge. She had figured her fear of men armed with weapons of war was a distant memory. Not so. That day in the bank, she told me, she again had become the little girl at her grandmother's side while uniformed men gave orders. The United States of America, the land that had provided asylum and opportunity now had stolen her sense of security. For two years, she and I examined that hidden pain that suddenly was brought to the present.

Yet it wasn't only that one SLA encounter or the thought of Japanese soldiers that had Mariana sitting across from me in my office. She had safely locked away memories of those very bad times. It was the several bank robberies she had endured as a teller.

Crocker Bank had acquired Hibernia, and Mariana kept her teller's job. Years later, she was robbed by a "big Black guy." It happened quickly. In and out. Was there a gun? "I did what I was supposed to. I handed over the bait money. I dropped the transponder in the bag. And as I gave this fellow the contents of my cash drawer, I heard him say, 'Don't do anything funny.' But I already had."

Mariana never saw the bank robber again, though she feared she might. But officers of the San Francisco Police Department told her they'd found the bait money and transponder in a public trash can two blocks from the bank. "He warned me!" Mariana told me. So, she waited for his return, for him to make good on his threat to make her pay for doing "anything funny." For a short time, the bank manager transferred her from the teller's window to a clerical position elsewhere in the bank lobby. Yet from her new desk, she could scan the customers coming through the door. And then it happened. "This Mexican fella robbed Phyllis right in front of me. The robber didn't pull a gun, so maybe the ordeal wasn't that bad," she said.

Several weeks later, Mariana was asked to return to a teller window. Though apprehensive, she didn't speak up – even though there were nightmares. At first, she worked half days behind a desk, away from customers, and half days at the teller's counter. Her co-worker, Phyllis, still had not returned to work, after doctor's orders to take a leave of absence. That option was never given to Mariana.

Mariana continued to show up for work, on time, praying that someday she'd be able to retire. Customers and co-workers, many of whom were years younger than she was, treated Mariana with respect. It was those other people, the strangers, who unnerved her.

"One weirdo after the next is what we deal with after the SSI checks are mailed each month," she told me. As the regulars mixed with the rabble, Mariana scanned the queue, looking for dark-skinned men who might be bank robbers. Her pulse would quicken when a Black man would approach her window. She once took an unscheduled bathroom break when she saw a Latino who looked like Phyllis' robber arguing with the security guard when he asked to examine a briefcase.

The blonde was well dressed, wearing the kind of pinstripe business suit that associates at pricey law firms wear. She waited patiently while Mariana finished up an account transaction. The woman in the suit handed Mariana a deposit slip but no check, no money, only a written message: "PUT THE LARGE BILLS IN AN ENVELOPE. KEEP SMILING. THIS IS NOT A JOKE. NOW."

This isn't right, thought Mariana. This person's not Black. Not a guy. Dressed like an attorney, an accountant, a bank auditor — not like a bank robber. "Excuse me, is there a problem?" It was the branch manager noticing something odd in Mariana's frozen appearance. She snapped to and assured the manager everything was in order. Meanwhile, the security guard was helping an older man with the door. The blonde slipped her right hand inside a handbag. Does she have a gun? If so, it's not needed. Mariana put the big bills into an envelope, about twenty 100s, two packets of 50s, and a bunch of 20s. Mariana asked, "Will there be anything else, ma'am?"

With her gloved left hand, the robber took the envelope and dropped it into the handbag. Then she placed her right hand into her handbag, brandished a silver handgun, and pointed it at Mariana's forehead. "Don't ever call me that, you old bitch." Then there was a distinctive click – but the gun did not fire. "Consider yourself lucky. My advice to you: Find another line of work," the blonde hissed. And then she was gone.

A few days later, Mariana and I met for the first time. She told me she hadn't been sleeping well. Her partner, George, would accompany her to my office for the next few weeks. She couldn't bring herself to venture out alone. Nothing seemed safe. Strangers weren't to be trusted, not even me, the doctor her employer recommended.

Treatment began with baby steps. It was not difficult to diagnose post-traumatic stress disorder (PTSD). PTSD became a diagnosis accepted by the American Psychiatric Association as a result of combat veterans returning from the Vietnam War and reliving life-threatening experiences such as firefights, ambushes, and mortar attacks. With Mariana, four bank robberies over a decade had left her reliving her terrors by day and struggling to sleep soundly at night. She found some relief from a sedating antidepressant that kept her from lying in bed, ruminating. When the fear of being out in public became too much, I prescribed an anti-anxiety drug to take the edge off. And we practiced relaxation techniques. With encouragement on my part, she would talk about the robberies. She also talked about the war. It became clear to me that she was beaten up and broken — but was willing to fight her demons.

Looking back, I could have done more for Mariana. I know she left treatment stronger yet still was troubled. Psychiatrists realize that outcomes for our patients are not the same sorts of outcomes that a doctor of another medical specialty seeks for their patients with appendicitis or a heart attack. Rarely is a patient with a mental problem "cured." For Mariana, there was no fix. She came to accept that she would not forget the traumas of her past. She stopped fearing and hating all strangers. But while she was able to venture into her neighborhood alone, she could not bring herself to return to the main bank branch where she was robbed, even in a position created for her that involved no contact with the public.

Ultimately, with the help of her attorney, Mariana negotiated a retirement package. But because she wanted her injury claim resolved quickly, the settlement was skimpy. No formal recognition from the employer for her years of service beyond a monthly check. Minimal acknowledgment of her sacrifice for continuing to work as a teller after the first three robberies. Nothing special was done for her. Mariana was not a complainer — she deserved more. And I should have fought for her. I realized that as an occupational psychiatrist, I sometimes also have to be a coach, an advocate, a resource, and much more.

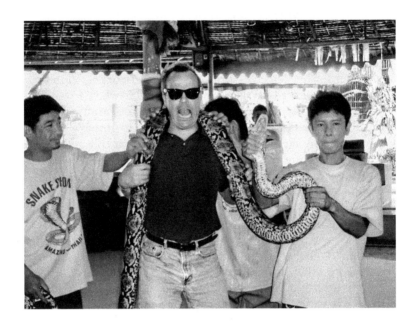

2 | Why Occupational Psychiatry?

No one starts out in life destined to become an occupational psychiatrist. In my experience, having listened to the life histories of thousands of people, very few knew at six, or eight, or ten what their career path would be. Certainly, some of the great concert pianists showed their potential and ability as a child. A few of the world's acclaimed painters demonstrated their gifts while in primary school. My wife knew which area of law she would practice before she entered middle school. I'm like most folks who tried something, had an opportunity present itself, and incrementally found myself.

I'm first-generation American on my mother's side. My mother, Emilia, was from Castel di Sangro ("Castle of Blood") in the Abruzzo region of Italy. She went to work at 14 when her father, who had been exposed to mustard gas while serving in the Italian army during World War I, could no longer work as a butcher. As a result, my mother never went to high school after coming to the United States at age eight. Em, as she would be called, worked 10-hour shifts, six days a week in a Chicago factory making various wheels to support her two parents and four younger brothers. Once she was married and had her own family, she wanted better for her kids. My brother and I were expected to do well in school. It was never a subject for debate. Later when I was in med school, my mom took night classes at the local community college and earned an associate's degree. She had something to prove.

No one in my family had ever graduated from college before me, followed by my younger brother, Guy (named after our grandfather Gitano). When I graduated from high school, I had no idea I would study medicine. I liked school. I didn't want to work in manufacturing plants like my folks. Still, I have fond memories as a boy accompanying my dad to the printing ink factory where he worked in the lab. The smells were warm and sweet. And there usually were girlie magazines lying around. Back then, the factory also produced adult literature along with the ink for other printing projects.

I grew up in the Sputnik era and had an excellent public school education. I learned some Latin at Sunday school and a little Italian at home. I signed up for French, but German and Russian were more suitable for a career in science. If you wanted to be a serious scientist, you were expected to read papers in English, German, and Russian. I also studied music, starting with the cornet and playing French horn into college. My brother and I were Mathletes in high school, though I was more nerdy yet less gifted than him. Guy could have become a math teacher or a professor. I was just a nerd. He was studying calculus and theoretical mathematics when most teens were memorizing things they would forget a week after taking their SAT.

Nerds apparently do OK in the long run, though there are no long-term outcome studies that prospectively follow nerds and captains of high school football teams. When I and the other fellow nerds roamed the halls of our high school, we didn't know that someday we would be pigeon-holed. There we were, holding our own against the jocks that the cool girls swooned over. Yep, we'd place our mechanical pencils ever so carefully in the pocket protectors of our white shirts. With our slide rules hanging on our belts, encased in real leather, we would fantasize about being gunslingers in a Wild West frontier town. Getting on the late afternoon bus with the football players and wrestlers was always a treat. I tried not to stumble when carrying my French horn case with my right hand while balancing a stack of chemistry texts and my chess set with my left arm. "Hey, Humpty, how'd the Word Problems do against Homewood last week?" (I'll explain how I got that nickname later.) Like my fellow nerds, I was a Mathlete and proud that Sandburg High was treated with respect by the math teams in our school's conference.

I still remember the weekend our school's science geeks visited the Illinois Institute of Technology. Wow, you could just imagine the experiments that undergrads got to be involved in at a technology institute! Maybe these guys even got to blow things up. There were similarities between us and a busload of Neanderthal jocks on the way to an athletic meet. Like the guys who played hoops and scored on the gridiron, we Mathletes went to competitions too, only our events challenged the organ residing between our tympanic membranes more than our muscles. Consider the slide rule competition, now a completely lost gladiator art form, where teams competed against the clock to solve complex calculations that determined who would reign as the fastest stick on any given Saturday.

Slide rules — kids today have no idea.

Then there were the word problems. Jody and Marian were all-star members of our crack team when it came to word problems. That's right: Mathletes, like the debate team, included male and female competitors on the same team! Girls could be nerds too, and some were shining stars, though few fantasized about blowing up stuff. And then there was Daryl, our secret weapon. "Come on, Daryl, do it." He could recite pi to at least 50 digits before most kids could spell Mississippi. He was a wiz. Daryl went on to earn a master's in theoretical mathematics before joining the accounting department of a Fortune 500 company.

During my freshman year at Carl Sandburg High School, word spread through the English department and into the far reaches of nerddom that auditions were taking place for "Alice in Wonderland," the spring play. I had some acting experience starring as Charlie Brown in a junior high production and had my sights set on the role of the Mad Hatter, which ultimately went to Tom, who charmed the audience.

Martha got the lead and did a fabulous job as Alice in her cute white blouse, navy skirt, and red pumps. (We'd take different paths only to end up at the same medical school and later in the same specialty.) No, I was destined to be Humpty Dumpty. It took a heroic effort to lower my voice as the oversized egg. And for the remainder of my high school years, I became known as "Humpty." Not just to tormenting jocks but to well-meaning teachers who somehow thought I took pride in having dressed up in tights and an eggshell costume for our community to laugh at as I fell off the wall, sometimes for two performances in a day. Three years later and with little regret, I left Humpty behind, when the University of Colorado (CU) located in Boulder entered my life and my acting career became a memory.

Whether due to fate or good fortune, another interest during my formative years led to studies at CU. After the famed Denver Zephyr transported my high school's concert band across the plains in passenger cars named Silver Bullet, Silver Legacy, Silver Shaft, and other variations of that precious metal, I found myself captivated by the Rocky Mountains. This was during the late 1960s, during the Vietnam War and civil rights movement, and those societal issues were the backdrop for a bunch of young teens on a great adventure. I still have photos of me goofing around with my friend Tom, who was first chair in the trumpet section. The music we played (mostly symphonic pieces or show tunes such as "Man of La Mancha" arranged for band) is a blur, but the exposure to the state of Colorado made a lasting impression. When it was time to apply to college, I submitted an application to CU.

That university changed my life. There's no way I would ever have taken a P.E. class in rock climbing at Northwestern or the University of Illinois. The million-volt electron microscope installed in CU's Department of Molecular, Cellular, and Developmental Biology would have a major impact on the path taken by this future occupational psychiatrist. My time at CU, plus years of training in medical school, a psychiatric residency, a master's program, and a health policy fellowship, provided the knowledge base to work clinically with emotionally troubled employees.

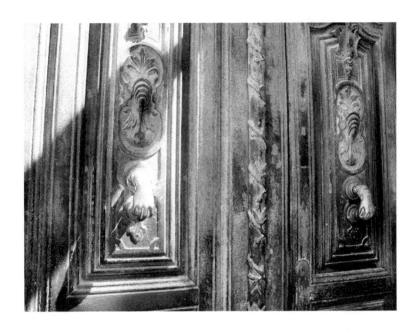

3 | Double Doors

I **knew there had to be some important secrets as the** professor opened the second of two doors to his office. He was a psychoanalyst and would be interviewing me for a residency program at the University of California, San Francisco (UCSF). His name was Dr. Mardi Horowitz, and he had authored the acclaimed textbook entitled, *Stress Response Syndrome.* I was not nervous meeting this preeminent PTSD clinical researcher. I had a good resume, strong letters of recommendation, and plenty of naiveté about the path on which I was embarking. Apparently, I made no horrible blunders as the program later offered me a position as a PGY-1 (first postgraduate year) intern-resident.

The view from the professor's office across Golden Gate Park was stunning. We must have talked about my reasons for considering the program based at the Langley Porter Psychiatric Institute (LLPI). We probably discussed my interest in psychiatry as a career. What I remember is his correcting me on using the term "instinct" about the mechanism used for self-reflection when making such a life choice. "Intuition is what you meant," he said. Of course, he was technically correct, but maybe there was a bit of the more basic drive operating as well. Horace Greeley had directed, "Go West, young man." That was my plan at the time. I had interviewed at the medical school of my alma mater in Denver. I was also making the rounds of programs in Albuquerque, Tucson, San Diego, Los Angeles, Portland and Seattle. Northwestern University in Chicago wanted me, but I had wanderlust. Dr. Horowitz noticed me staring at the park beyond his office. He accurately noted, "You're smitten." He was right. I passed back through those double doors at the conclusion of our meeting thinking of another time when great and wondrous secrets had awaited me through a set of doors some five years earlier.

I took a work-study job during my sophomore year in Boulder. The Molecular, Cellular & Developmental Biology department was full of scientists, postdoctoral fellows, and PhD candidates. A few lucky undergrads snagged jobs working in molecular, cellular, and developmental biology. Exciting stuff. Dr. Goldstein's lab was dedicated to studying a particular unicellular organism, Amoeba proteus. I learned basic lab techniques. My initial duties included sterilizing glassware, collecting radioactive waste, and keeping the supplies in neat order. I was never asked to fetch coffee for the professor or pick up a researcher's lunch. I was treated with respect by my co-workers though Dr. Goldstein made clear his assessment of me. "Robert, you are the most absent-minded lab assistant I have ever employed. It would behoove you to keep reminders of tasks left unfinished." I thought it was a bit harsh to be labeled as forgetful, but to this day, I keep a to-do list in my shirt pocket.

Over time, I was given more-complex assignments related to research. One means by which scientists study cells is through the use of microscopes. To do so requires preserving biological matter. Unlike the crude fixatives used by anatomists or taxidermists, cell biologists use more-powerful agents. Instead of hydrocarbons such as formaldehyde, which stink, our lab used osmium tetroxide. Having worked with volatile chemicals, such as toluene for W. R. Grace and Company in Chicago before and after my freshman year, I had developed respect for the toxic effect of such compounds. But in Dr. Goldstein's lab, the work was more intense. The chemicals we worked with had to be handled carefully under ventilated hoods. The form of liquid osmium we used came in small, glass ampoules. After breaking the glass open, the cells or tissue are then placed in the liquid osmium, which turns live stuff

10

into rock. If you can smell the osmium, your brain is being fixated, and you're about to die. That was dangerous and scary stuff to work around for the princely sum of $4.25 an hour. Needless to say, I never made a mistake working with osmium tetroxide.

My work in the lab led to my assisting Dr. Gary Wise, a postdoc. Gary had earned his doctorate at the University of California at Berkeley before moving to Boulder. We got along famously. Because I helped to prepare samples for study, Gary invited me into the microscopy suite one day. The preserved tissue had been encased in epoxy, sliced with a diamond microtome, and then placed onto miniscule, thin gold wafers. Once placed on discs using the most delicate of tweezers, the material was ready for examination with a million-volt electron microscope, reached via an air lock. The interview with Dr. Horowitz required me to go through a similar set of double doors some years later and reminded me of the wonders I was exposed to at CU. When Gary cranked up the magnification of the microscope, we were taken inside the cell. It felt like we were landing on the moon. The mystery of life is amazing, whether a cell, a lunar surface, or the human psyche.

For me, getting hooked on cell biology was easy. Dr. Keith Porter was the chair of our department in Boulder. He had written the leading textbook on cell biology, which incorporated photos taken with electron microscopes to illustrate the structure of cells. Nuclei, mitochondria, and ribosomes are much more enticing as sharp black-and-white images rather than just descriptions in a paragraph. While learning the science of cellular life and the techniques for probing inside viruses and amoeba, I was also exposed to debates over the war in Vietnam, nuclear energy, and the Equal Rights Amendment. The 1970s was a time of exploration of much more than the inside of unicellular organisms. I learned that scientists are not apolitical and certainly enjoy voicing their opinions. Dr. Goldstein seemed more excited by seeing his letter to the editor published in The New York Times on the war and its repercussions, than when his peer-reviewed article on incorporating an organism's structure entirely as a new intracellular body was accepted by a scientific publication.

Along with my lab duties, I picked up enough basic knowledge to assume the role of teaching assistant while still an undergrad myself. This was in classrooms using light microscopes with fellow students who were expected to study life firsthand, not by memorizing facts in texts. In those settings, I came to think critically of "premeds." They were students who, by my assessment, didn't really love studying and learning, but instead challenged themselves to retain information, do well at multiple choice tests, and to dream of giving orders in a hospital. Meanwhile, they were seemingly unaware of the opportunities all around them. These premeds projected themselves forward to a time when they would be real doctors — while often missing out on the beauty of knowledge and of systems across disciplines. God forbid one might actually find Picasso, Einstein, or Jefferson to be thought provoking.

Looking back, I realize that double doors are not simply a physical barrier but also are a metaphor. In the literal sense, they represent a barrier to germs. Metaphorically, they stand for a secret hiding place. There are germs and dirt particles that invade bodies and degrade biological samples. Some thoughts should be safeguarded if an individual is to feel safe in disclosing the truth and becoming vulnerable to the input of a psychoanalyst. We not only learn about the life of the microbes we explore with electron microscopes and tissue culture, we test ourselves by attempting to solve the puzzle of life. Do mental health practitioners test themselves, while unlocking the secrets of our fellow humans, when they come to us as patients suffering from our shared existence? In the next chapter, you will learn of a confrontational clinical approach I developed as a means to delve into secrets and to change selfish behavior in the business community.

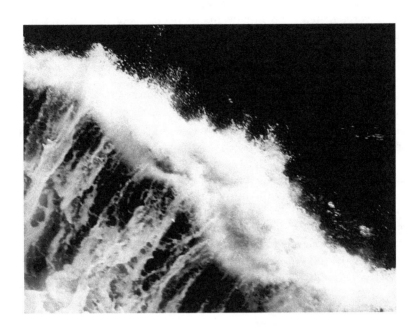

4 | Slapping Therapy

One thing that attracted me to the training program at UCSF was the eclectic nature of the four years of study required of psychiatric residents. The first year was an internship evenly split between medicine and psychiatry assignments in hospitals. Each medicine rotations lasted a month: emergency room, neurology, two general medical inpatient rotations, Cancer Research Institute (CRI), and the Kidney Transplant Unit (KTU). My neurology training was at San Francisco General Hospital (SFGH), the county hospital.

Occasionally, we were fortunate to have an instructor who could really teach, and that turned out to be the case for me at SFGH. Rather than putting every patient through the same mental status exam, we were expected to find a topic of interest for each patient as a means to explore potential deficits in mentation. If my patient was a Giants baseball fan, I wouldn't ask him who the last five presidents of the United States were. Instead, I'd pursue his recollection of how his team did against the dreaded Dodgers. Unlike my experience at Northwestern during medical school, you could not expect that a patient admitted to neurology was primarily suffering from a nervous system disorder. At times, a new patient admitted from the ER would turn out to have a gastrointestinal bleed as the cause for reduced consciousness, not a head injury. So, it was a good learning experience — as long as the patient lived. Things aren't always what they appear to be. And shrinks are supposed to think like "real doctors."

My assignments to the ER and medical wards went by with no trauma, to the doctor. Which means I felt up to the task, and no patient was injured, much less killed. You're expected to take things seriously when you sign on as one's physician. If you don't, become a standup comic or a radio talk show host. I was diligent and felt I was in a good groove. Then came the KTU, the Kidney Transplant Unit at UCSF. In the mid-1970s, it was the busiest transplant service in America. It was a "med-surg" ward where the medicine interns had responsibility for keeping patients from rejecting their new organs. As surgeons say, "To cut is to cure." This means the other physicians, nurses, and health-care personnel had to make sure the postop patient didn't die. It was a tough job to prevent infection, transplant rejection, and hemorrhaging. I found myself up to the task. It's not work for the timid, and it usually results in young interns becoming adult doctors.

If the KTU was a challenge akin to hiking the Appalachian Trail, the Cancer Research Institute was like climbing Mount Everest without oxygen. Who in their right mind thought future psychiatrists should be writing doctor's orders for patients admitted to a tertiary care facility who had failed chemotherapy trials at multiple other hospitals? These folks weren't just sick; they were dying. And they weren't expected to die in years or decades, but months, weeks, or days. We lost patients every day. For young men and women staffing the service as nurses and doctors, it was a brutal assignment. The nurses were truly like nuns or perhaps saints. The interns and residents rotated off the service of death, while the nurses stayed and lent continuity and hope to those who returned for a second or third round of high-tech poison.

My dad had been a medic in World War II, assigned to a unit in Burma, so a few weeks into my CRI experience, I phoned home. I told him I hadn't been away from the ward for even one day. When I wasn't on call, I was studying treatment protocols or driving to San Francisco International Airport to pick up blood products flown in for a patient. I recall my father saying, "So what's the problem?" To which I responded, "I'm afraid I'm going to kill someone." Not uncommonly,

I would administer chemo in one vein, which resulted in immune suppression and the need to use two additional IVs to deliver packed cells and antibiotics. Death was a very real prospect for my charges. "Quit feeling sorry for yourself. For Christ's sake, you're not the poor bastard with lung cancer." Dad told me. "You're well trained, and these people need you. So, get back to work, and save someone."

Experiences in the KTU and the CRI dealing with life and death, as well as my later handling psychiatric emergencies, helped me to develop "slapping therapy." For five years, I had a part-time position with the psychiatric emergency service at Highland General Hospital (HGH), the county hospital for Oakland. Well, you get to see extreme personal catastrophes working a 24-hour shift at HGH. I started moonlighting there during the third year of my residency. I had already had jobs in a clinic in the Tenderloin District of San Francisco, doing histories and physicals on inpatients at a psychiatric facility in the East Bay, and making visits to board and care facilities in East Oakland. I was good at making command decisions on patients with complicated medical and psychiatric problems.

At the Langley Porter Psychiatric Institute (LPPI) of UCSF, the residents shared a call schedule covering the medical center for any psychiatric emergencies and consultations, aside from admitting patients to the psychiatric hospital. In one night at LPPI, a resident might admit two patients and consult on another. At HGH, the psychiatrist on duty might have more than 20 new cases show up during a work shift: drug overdoses cleared by the medical ER, paranoid schizophrenics brought in by the Oakland Police Department for walking naked down East 14th Street, a borderline personality having made his fourth suicide attempt in the two weeks since his lover left him, or a family man depressed about having no money for Christmas after losing his job at the local auto plant. These were people who needed care at HGH. We learned to work quickly and efficiently.

※ ※ ※ ※ ※ ※ ※ ※ ※ ※ ※ ※ ※ ※ ※

Years later in private practice, I developed a consultative relationship with a Big Eight accounting firm. The vice president for human resources would turn to our medical group when dealing with a particularly difficult employee. A typical scenario involved an international tax law expert who was technically superb but was a moron working with others. Similar to my father's blunt style of getting to the heart of things, I would conduct slapping therapy.

Dr. Bob: "So why do you think the head of HR referred you to a psychiatrist?"
Accountant: "I'm not sure."

Dr. Bob:	"OK. Do you think it might have anything to do with how you get along with people?"
Accountant:	"What people?"
Dr. Bob:	"Let's start with secretaries. How many personal secretaries have been assigned to you in the last year?"
Accountant:	"I don't know, probably a few."
Dr. Bob:	"It's been five."
Accountant:	"Fine. And your point is what?"
Dr. Bob:	"My point is that your last executive secretary, administrative assistant or however you'd refer to her, is more valuable to the company that employs the two of you than you are."
Accountant:	"Bulls***."
Dr. Bob:	"She's been with the accounting firm since you were in kindergarten. She gave you six months' notice before a two-week vacation. She came to work with her bags packed expecting to work through the afternoon and then catch her flight to Paris. And then at 4 p.m. you dropped a three-hour transcription on her desk, telling her to, 'Get it done right away'."
Accountant:	"Well, the client was pleased."
Dr. Bob:	"Yes, and your co-worker's vacation was wrecked. She demanded a transfer, like a long line of employees who want nothing to do with you. So here's the deal. You change or you're gone."
Accountant:	"Who do you think you are? I don't have to put up with your attitude."
Dr. Bob:	"No, you don't. But if you want to make partner and not be unemployed, you'll have to change your attitude."
Accountant:	"I can't afford to lose this position. I've been with the firm for six years. I can't just start over."
Dr. Bob:	"Then you have a problem. Would you like my help in trying to work things out?"
Accountant:	"I guess so."
Dr. Bob:	"All right. I'll give you three more sessions to show me that your co-workers are as valuable as your clients' bank accounts. Think about it. I'll see you next week at this same time if that works for you."
Accountant:	"OK. See you then."
Dr. Bob:	"One more thing. I have a homework assignment for you. I understand you have a new administrative assistant working for you. I'd like you to tell me two ways you welcomed her to that relationship over the next week. Because your reputation precedes you. Good luck."

At our second session, the accountant was on time and smiling. He could barely contain his desire to report the good news.

Accountant: "Her name is Sally, and I think she likes me."
Dr. Bob: "Who is Sally?"
Accountant: "My admin person. See, I know her name."
Dr. Bob: "OK. That's good. How did you welcome her?"
Accountant: "I took the time to say, 'Good morning. How are you today?'"
Dr. Bob: "Nice. How did she respond?"
Accountant: "She said she was fine and thanked me for asking."
Dr. Bob: "Anything else to report?"
Accountant: "Yep. I came back from lunch with a bouquet of flowers that I presented to her. I then asked her if she had the time to help me with a report for a client that needed to get out that day."
Dr. Bob: "And her reaction was what?"
Accountant: "She seemed surprised by the flowers and said she could work on the report once she got the flowers in some water. We knocked out the report, and before she left that day, Sally made a point of saying, 'Have a nice night.'"
Dr. Bob: "What was that whole experience like for you?"
Accountant: "It made me feel decent. I had so much energy I went for a long run after getting home from downtown."
Dr. Bob: "Looks like you might get it, like you may be able to change when you put effort into doing so."

This is slapping therapy. The patient is confronted with reality. There is limited confidentiality. Someone else is paying the bill. Someone else is interested in the outcome. There is an avenue to corroborate the patient's account of how things go in the workplace. There is a carrot and a big stick. I am the facilitator. I help those who are ready to see reality. As good as you are, in some ways, there are parts of you that must adapt. If not, you will have to start over, somewhere else. And probably for much less money. The slap can wake up the future partner who goes on to work cooperatively with others. It also might have no effect on the asocial jerk. Slapping therapy is just one component of the occupational psychiatrist's armamentarium.

$\wp\!\!\sim\!\!\wp\!\!\sim\!\!\wp\!\!\sim\!\!\wp\!\!\sim\!\!\wp\!\!\sim\!\!\wp\!\!\sim\!\!\wp\!\!\sim\!\!\wp\!\!\sim\!\!\wp\!\!\sim\!\!\wp\!\!\sim\!\!\wp$

Not infrequently, I am referred an individual who is exceedingly thin-skinned. This is an ordinary person who has been blessed with good health, born into a family with two loving parents, and has never faced a serious challenge. But something unexpected presents itself, and the world seems to fall apart for Mr. Ordinary. He assumes a victim role, and the focus of his existence becomes "Why me?" Please. Such members of our species consume tremendous resources while regressing to a childlike stance where they are cared for by family, health professionals, and the greater society. I am not speaking of people who have been in life-threatening situations. I'm speaking of those who have experienced an accident or hardship that creates only temporary discomfort. And slapping therapy would not make a difference.

A fellow named John comes to mind. He was laid off from his job as an appliance salesman for a national retailer following a corporate acquisition. He'd been with the company long enough to get a buyout package. Three months later, he was offered a sales manager opportunity with a competitor. Though he acknowledged his good fortune, he couldn't let go of the slight of being dumped by the predecessor. John's primary care physician referred him to our practice. His symptoms were largely psychosomatic — heartburn and headaches. He was also consumed by his anger for the former HR manager who picked him as part of the group to be laid off. Slapping therapy began in our third session when he was confronted with the reality that many people he knew were less fortunate yet complained less than he did. John's narcissism prevented him from appreciating either the suffering or the resilience of others. I realized it would take a far more serious life event for him to even consider changing his ways. Slapping therapy would be of little use. Character pathology that is well established is not easily given up.

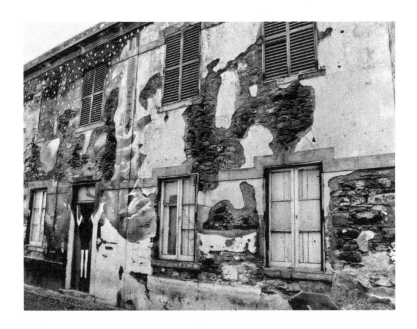

5 | House Calls

Psychiatrists and other physicians don't usually make house calls. They treat patients in an office. But over the years, I have made home visits or house calls.

In 1977, I spent six weeks in an externship through the Department of Psychiatry at the University of New Mexico (UNM) School of Medicine in Albuquerque. That experience counted toward my clinical requirements as a medical student at Northwestern. During that month and a half, I shared a small house on two acres not far from the Rio Grande. I was assigned to tag along with instructors in the Indian Mental Health program. That included visiting homes of Native Americans in Bernalillo County. One of those visits stands out.

It was a warm afternoon when a professor of psychiatry and I drove up to the very modest adobe home in a semi-rural section of Albuquerque, some distance from downtown and the UNM Medical Center. We were greeted outside by a 45-year-old Pueblo Indian named Johnny. He was expecting us. His fenced-in yard was mostly gravel and weeds. Two dogs lay in the shade. I followed Johnny through his wide-open front door. I took a seat in a wooden chair with arms in a simple living room.

I was introduced to Johnny as a visiting medical student who would be listening in on the session. I had read through his chart the night before and on the drive over had discussed his case with my professor. Johnny had been in and out of psychiatric hospitals over the previous 20 years for episodes of psychosis and substance abuse involving alcohol and amphetamines. The prior year, he had completed a drug treatment program and remained sober while regularly attending Alcoholics Anonymous meetings. For the last six months, he had been living alone in the tiny house his family owned. He wasn't working but remained involved in the pueblo where he had grown up. He was welcome to participate in dances performed by men of the kiva that he first entered with his father as a boy.

Johnny told us he didn't like to travel to the medical center or even to a clinic close to his home. We were visiting him to make sure he was taking his medication. We also were interested in seeing how he was taking care of himself. I recall that he was in a pleasant mood. He had received notice that his application for Social Security disability benefits had been approved, which meant he would no longer have to depend on assistance from his family. He showed us his pill bottles containing an antipsychotic drug and a mood stabilizer. He took them twice a day, as instructed, he told us, and he no longer needed Antabuse to maintain sobriety. Over the past week, he had attended three 12-step meetings. He denied hearing voices or having evil thoughts.

I had never been to a house with dirt floors. While there was some order to it, it was dusty. The windows needed cleaning. The living quarters weren't my style, but things seemed orderly. Indian baskets hung on a wall, and a bookcase held clay pots typical of those fashioned at his pueblo. He had a pot of beans cooking in the kitchen. It smelled good. I was feeling comfortable with our visit when Johnny interrupted my professor and said, "You might want to tell the boy there's a snake under his chair." I saw the doctor look toward me and become silent. I was aware that at times, Johnny had been delusional. He also had a reputation as a jokester, according to his chart. That didn't make him a liar. Rather than show disdain for his warning by sliding my feet under my chair, I bent over to peek. To my surprise, a large Western diamondback was coiled there and gazing at me. Its good-sized rattle was silent.

Using the arms of the chair, I levitated, with my feet coming to rest on the seating surface of the chair. Johnny stood up, went outside, and returned with a shovel. He walked straight at me and bent down to scoop up the rattler. After turning toward the doorway, he passed my professor, who remained silent. He tossed the snake into the yard. "I've been trying to get that fellow all morning," he stated. The session ended within minutes, and I have no memory of what else took place. That visit to Johnny's home was certainly unlike any consultation that might take place back home in Chicago.

ഏ൚ഏ൚ഏ൚ഏ൚ഏ൚ഏ൚ഏ൚ഏ൚ഏ൚ഏ൚ഏ൚

A few years later, after my stint in Albuquerque, I again would make home visits to provide mental health services to the chronically mentally ill. During my residency training at the LPPI in San Francisco, I "moonlighted" at part-time jobs. A psychiatrist, Dr. Jim Liles, who had completed the same residency program was now in practice in Oakland. He offered me a position to occasionally see patients in his offices, but more regularly to visit board and care homes in Oakland and neighboring communities.

These homes were in working-class neighborhoods. Each had a resident manager or owner who looked after a household of adults with histories of mental illness. Common diagnoses were schizophrenia, bipolar disorder, major depression, and borderline personality disorder. The homes usually housed four to six residents. The larger homes kept both men and women. These places were intended to provide shelter for patients who no longer needed to be hospitalized yet could not live independently.

My role was to visit the homes to make sure the residents were getting by without the need for a more structured setting, i.e., a hospital. At each home, I got to know the manager, any staff, and the residents. The managers would inform me of any tantrums or episodes of acting out. Decisions were made about adjusting the dosage of medication, using timeouts, and referring cantankerous patients to a locked facility where aggressive behavior could be better managed.

Some homes were actually homey. They typically had an owner who was compassionate and understanding. Most of the managers and owners I visited had minimal training. Obtaining a license to operate a home for a mentally ill population was not difficult as it was in the state's interest to get these troubled souls out of hospitals, for cost reasons. This resulted in some owners having multiple homes and hiring staff to look after their residents. In those situations, it was sometimes a challenge to differentiate the staff from the patients. Some staff treated residents like children, or worse, as criminals. I came to know which managers and staffs were likely to use medication to either punish or intentionally

21

sedate their residents. Suffice it to say that in the year I made home visits as a psychiatrist, I learned a lot about how life is for those who suffer from serious mental illness in America.

ട്ട്ട്ട്ട്ട്ട്ട്ട്ട്ട്ട്ട്ട്ട്ട്ട്

Occasionally in my role as an evaluating psychiatrist, I am asked to consult in an individual's home. While I prefer not to work with men and women who are incarcerated, I have occasionally performed consultations in prisons or state hospitals. These institutions are "homes" for the inmates they house. One time I visited San Quentin State Prison to meet with a prisoner for an injury claim that predated his incarceration. San Quentin is in a truly lovely setting in Marin County — with its spectacular views of San Francisco and Alcatraz. It's also spooky. When you visit such a facility, you are informed by the guards that should a hostage situation develop, the authorities will not negotiate for your release. Needless to say, I was exceedingly efficient in conducting the assessment of the claimant and found no reason to return to the prison for a second session.

On another occasion, I met with a resident of Atascadero State Hospital to evaluate the merits of a work-related injury claim that predated this man's hospitalization. Atascadero is a psychiatric facility that houses the criminally insane. Many of the patients there could have ended up in prison or are ex-felons. The hospital is situated among the rolling hills of central California. The setting is idyllic. Don't be fooled. The facility contains some exceedingly dangerous people. The staff must remain constantly vigilant. Under such circumstances, I review pertinent records beforehand and know what questions to ask. I don't rush the assessment, but I don't spend much time in chitchat. Again, I don't plan to return.

There are other evaluations where the subject genuinely cannot go to a doctor's office. That's because these cases involve persons with well-documented histories of severe anxiety. Some are terrified to fly. Some fear heights, which prevents them crossing bridges. With these sorts of people, I go to the city where they live, and we meet in a professional setting, such as a medical or law office.

ട്ട്ട്ട്ട്ട്ട്ട്ട്ട്ട്ട്ട്ട്ട്ട്ട്

Many years after my home visits in Albuquerque, I was asked to conduct an interview in a claimant's home. After reading through the file, I agreed to do so. This was a tragic case of a death of a construction laborer working near the San Francisco International Airport. A death claim had been settled with the family of the deceased. Mr. Olson was the project manager at that worksite. He was a highly experienced professional in his mid-50s with no history of emotional problems. And he now held himself responsible for the young man's death. He had instructed the laborer to dig a hole. But nearby was a backhoe driven by a heavy equipment operator unaware of the laborer's presence. The backhoe struck the laborer in the head resulting in death. A Cal/OSHA investigation found no wrongdoing on Mr. Olson's part. In retrospect, a series of mistakes occurred, but there was no finding of negligence.

In the weeks and months that followed the man's death, Mr. Olson began taking more and more time away from the construction project he oversaw. At the request of his employer, he met with his regular physician, who placed him on a leave. A replacement was found to complete the project. Time went by, and Mr. Olson became increasingly reclusive. He had been living alone since his wife's death two years earlier. Company representatives became concerned after visiting him in his home. A referral was made for him to meet with a treating psychiatrist near his home. Treatment was instituted, which included the prescriptions of an antidepressant and an anti-anxiety drug. On multiple dates, the manager missed scheduled appointments — because he had developed obsessive compulsive symptoms and agoraphobia for venturing out of his home.

It had been more than a year since the laborer's death when Mr. Olson and I met at his home. It was neat and tidy. He could afford the services of a housekeeper and a landscaping crew. He was well groomed and polite. He continued in treatment with his psychiatrist. Sessions with that physician were monthly. Mr. Olson continued to take psychotropic (psychiatric) medication. He had gotten a dog at the suggestion of his psychiatrist and walked the pet in his neighborhood. He used a grocery delivery service. His employer had tried to accommodate him by letting him work from home on contracts and project planning.

Ultimately, Mr. Olson and his long-term employer agreed that it would be best if he retired. Financially, he had no worries. But to me, he was a sad and troubled soul unable to forgive himself for the worker's death. More-intensive counseling had been suggested, but he made it clear he was not interested. Through legal counsel, he had asked that his work-related psychiatric injury claim, filed by his employer, be settled. There was insufficient reason to institute treatment on an involuntary basis. He was not a danger to himself or others, nor was he gravely disabled and unable to care for himself. My report guaranteed that Mr. Olson would receive an award for lifetime psychiatric care. It was not a particularly satisfying outcome for the last house call made by this psychiatrist.

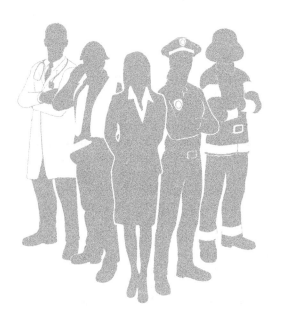

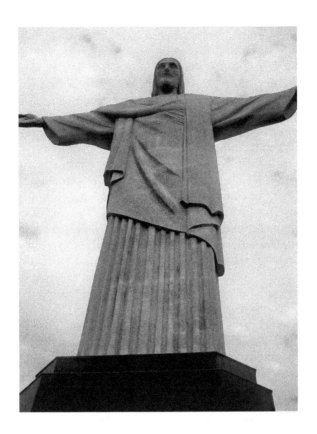

6 | What Does Not Kill Me Makes Me Stronger

Not all trauma victims remain victims. Not all those subjected to robbery, violence, and repeated abuse develop PTSD. Some have symptoms of an acute stress response, such as intense fear, insomnia, and startle reactions, but these unwelcome features dissipate in weeks or months, and a chronic disorder never develops. Like Mariana, whose story was depicted in Chapter One, Ben, another trauma victim, visited us in our offices. He should best be viewed as someone who developed "post-traumatic growth" (PTG).

PTG as a trauma response is analogous to developing a bolstered immune system after becoming infected with a virulent pathogen: "What does not kill me makes me stronger." For assistant managers of fast-food restaurants raped when making a night deposit, long-term airline employees laid off for no fault of their own, and farm workers subjected to amputation by machinery, emotional turmoil is a common response. Not uncommonly, clinicians tell patients that what they are experiencing is "normal." Common, normal, expected, but not right, and very uncomfortable. So how much solace can one take in being told that intrusive thoughts of a rape are expected? How helpful is it to a flight attendant to learn it's common to avoid air travel while furloughed? Does a farm worker amputee find comfort in gaining an understanding that it's normal to dream about still having both arms? A normal response to trauma is not a state of health — but is what happens after a serious trauma or loss. Assisting those exposed to trauma to come to an understanding about what is to be expected is part of the job of a mental health worker. Psychoeducation is the process of helping the patient to know what to expect after the initial trauma has passed.

※ ❧ ※ ❧ ※ ❧ ※ ❧ ※ ❧ ※ ❧ ※ ❧ ※ ❧ ※ ❧ ※ ❧ ※ ❧

An example: Ben was a battalion chief for a small firehouse in rural Northern California. His normal duties involved managing the firehouse, including equipment and personnel, while working a 24-hour shift. He also was expected to assess large scale fires via aerial surveillance while flying in small airplanes or helicopters. He studied forestry in college and took pride in his work as a professional firefighter. He knew he was good at what he did and expected those around him to show a similar commitment to excellence.

Fire season in California historically peaks in the late summer and early fall, when the earth is parched and the timber dry. A fire of more than 10,000 acres was blazing when Ben got the call that his services were needed. On this occasion, he went up in a helicopter with a young pilot and a spotter. While ascending over a ridge, the helicopter clipped the top of a tree and crashed. The pilot and spotter were thrown clear. Ben came to in the wreckage. His left leg was broken in multiple places. A disc in his lower back was herniated. The metal structure of the chopper came to rest upon him. He knew he was bleeding profusely. To his horror, he realized he was covered in aviation fuel, while the wildfire was making its way up the hillside. If he was to die on this hillside, he prayed he would bleed out before the flames reached him.

A group of firefighters had seen the crash. They dropped their personal safety equipment and charged up the slope to rescue their comrades. The pilot and spotter were not seriously injured and represented no extraction problem for the firefighters. Once carefully removed from the wreckage, Ben was strapped to a stretcher. The team took turns carrying him, at great peril to themselves, to a site from which they could all be evacuated. Once Medevac'd to a trauma center, it took 20 units of blood products to stabilize Ben. A metal rod was implanted in his left leg at the site of multiple femoral fractures. The ruptured disc was removed, and one level of his spine was fused. He had to learn to walk again. The opiates that kept his pain in check also led to addiction. And through a long recovery, Ben became obsessed with one thought. KILL THE PILOT!

What tormented Ben was learning that the copter pilot never should have been on that mission. His flight history had been misrepresented. He did not have the requisite experience to fly into a massive conflagration. He had not heeded the instructions, given before takeoff, to dump or burn off fuel because of conditions present. As a result, the aircraft was too heavy and could not produce sufficient lift to clear the tree line. Because of the crash, Ben had come close to death, and his life would never be the same.

Ben learned who the pilot was and became obsessed. He fumed about the arrogance of the man who caused this preventable accident. He contemplated revenge. Would it be a slow, torturous death or a maiming that would leave the young man disfigured and in chronic pain, awaiting his eventual passing? Would a gun, a knife, or a sledge hammer be used? These fantasies gave Ben pleasure as he projected the hell that would befall the man responsible for his misery.

Understand that these morbid fantasies were taking place in the mind of a man with no history of violence or antisocial tendencies. Ben was angry and depressed. Those who knew him saw the change in his demeanor. Eventually, his wife confronted him and made it clear that she could no longer share his hate-filled existence. She managed to get through to Ben.

Call it an "Aha!" moment. Or perhaps it was an epiphany. One and a half years after the crash, Ben realized that if he were ever to fully heal, he would have to forgive the pilot. Was it a spiritual awakening in a man not particularly religious? Ben took steps to accept the traumatic event and its outcome. His daily use of opiates was tapered off, and he eventually discontinued them. He started venturing out from the room in which he had cloistered himself. He looked into returning to work and found himself welcomed when he did so.

This story of tragedy and redemption was painful. Ben is left with chronic pain and significant physical limitations. He gets dejected and finds himself feeling "tight" when learning of fellow first responders being in harm's way. But he also has a renewed appreciation for life. He's an example of a man who was traumatized but does not remain a victim. He travels more with his spouse. He is closer to his adult son. He has renewed his interest in black-and-white photography. He teaches and mentors younger firefighters. Because of the resilience, or mettle, he has demonstrated, Ben was recognized with the Courage Award given by the California Society of Industrial Medicine and Surgery: it's given to an injured worker who has shown remarkable perseverance in returning to the workforce after serious trauma. Not all victims remain victims.

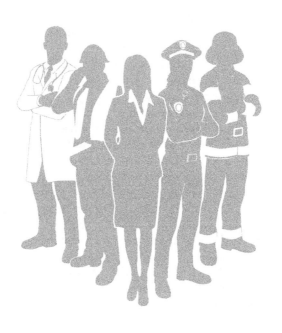

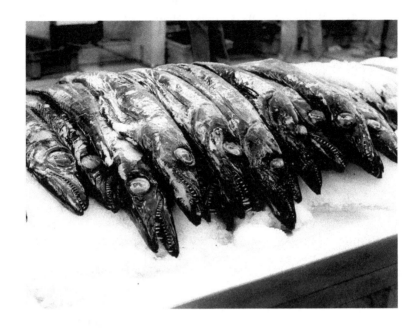

7 | The Psychological Autopsy

Many of us are raised believing it's impolite to discuss the circumstances of a person's death. This is especially true with suicides. There are legal reasons, however, when it is necessary to investigate how and why a person has died. A psychological autopsy might take place when the circumstances of an individual's death are obscure. For me, raised by an Italian mother whose culture did not shy away from the topic of death, this type of investigation perhaps fits well with my personality.

Growing up in the Midwest in the early 1960s, winter would at times bring "snow days" where a storm left enough white wonder that schools were closed for a day or two while the plows cleared the roadways. Even for kids who enjoyed class time, these were welcome occasions to spend unstructured time with neighbors. Building snow forts, sledding down hillsides, and engaging in snowball fights can easily occupy a day. I recall the stillness, the quiet, and the icicles hanging from gutters. Usually there were chores, such as shoveling the sidewalk or the driveway. No snow blowers, just gloves, and a snow shovel. Then another snowball fight before going inside, where dinner was cooking and more chores awaited. Time to set up the tray tables before Dad got home. We'd eat pasta and peas while listening to Walter Cronkite. Some nights it was Huntley and Brinkley. This was the early 1960s.

There were other ways to get out of school. A bad cold might work. I never did anything bad enough to get suspended, though that seemed to get some classmates a reprieve from English, math, and social studies. A serious illness in the family necessitating a hospital visit could justify a day away from academics as well. My personal favorite was funerals. An entire day would be spent for some old person's memorial. I liked it best when I didn't know the dead fellow. My brother, Guy, and I would accompany our mom on these occasions while Dad went to work. We'd dress up and travel to a Catholic church for Mass, and it wasn't even Sunday! Then a procession of vehicles would follow the hearse to the cemetery, where the priest would talk some more. Crying would occur. Lots of flowers would be left at the gravesite.

Finally, you'd end up at someone's home where a wake would be held with tons of Italian food to eat. Boys and girls got to drink red wine. Stories about the deceased, some scary and some funny, were told for hours. I remember meeting an aunt who apparently hated cats. She lived in a tall brownstone apartment building that had a breezeway, her favorite place to drop bricks while trying to kill felines. That aunt never married, for good reason.

So, death was a part of my upbringing. It wasn't hidden. It was part of life. Sometimes sad, sometimes creepy, but never were children excluded from knowing it had visited. While still a teenager, I learned that a former classmate from high school had died. That was different. Rusty jumped to his death during his freshman year at college. That was beyond sad. Later, while working at two major medical centers in Miami and Boston, I began to get routinely exposed to deaths of young and old. Deaths caused by accident, illness, gunshots, toxins, quarrels, beatings, exposure, drugs, and other hazards, both modern and ancient. The departments I worked in as a lab tech had county morgues, so bodies were ever present. I didn't participate in autopsies, but I was aware they were taking place. I was exposed to the gallows humor of the pathologists. It was some years later that I would find myself conducting psychological autopsies.

A tradition in medical training of the 20th century required first year medical school students to spend a year immersed in the subject of Gross Anatomy. For some of us trainees, it was clear why the term "gross" applied. I had studied microbiology as an undergraduate only to find myself and three peers spending long hours dissecting a cadaver. We named the body Hector. He was a thin, older fellow. I don't think we ever figured out what led to his demise. Toward the end of the academic year, Hector was literally sinew and bones. The formaldehyde used as an embalming agent kept the tissue moist, but with time, and as a result of exploration with probes and hands, he began to appear less and less human. And the smell of the preservative saturated not only our lab coats but invaded our clothing and even our skin. In those seemingly ancient times, students did not use gloves, so the chemicals that drenched our hands would cause temporary numbness. Often, fellow bus passengers of the Chicago Transit Authority would notice the sweet smell of the hydrocarbons that identified med students heading home for the night as some type of modern-day ghouls.

I met my good friend Mark when he sat in with my anatomy team on Day One of our life with Hector. Mark was not as disgusted by the process of cutting up a body as I was, though he struggled with the memorization, as did most of us not destined to be surgeons. We devised an analog system in which we tagged and labeled nerves, muscles, and blood vessels. I got Mark through the year of anatomy and he'd pay me back when we started cutting on live specimens.

Ironically, years later it turned out that three members of Hector's team chose the field of psychiatry. As with Mark and Emily, there was no way to predict that I, a working-class kid, would opt for the specialty area identified with Freud. Yet it came to pass. As a result of the path chosen, a most unique procedure became part of my professional existence: the psychological autopsy.

Forensic psychiatrists typically examine live subjects. However, there are situations where the subject is deceased, yet the circumstances are such that questions persist. Was death by suicide? If so, what was the dynamic issue driving the deceased to act in a mortal manner? Some legal jurisdictions require an answer to the inquiry, "Was there an irresistible impulse?" You would be mistaken to assume it's all rather obvious. Most of the time, it is. Not always. Medical records and police reports are reviewed. Unfortunately, family members are commonly interviewed. There's nothing worse than asking probative questions of a spouse desperate to receive death benefits from an insurer if suicide is supported by the facts. Sometimes a guy dies when a loved one who was expected to be the rescuer comes home late. Too bad, she pulled an extra shift at the manufacturing plant and no one was there to find him after another overdose. S*** happens.

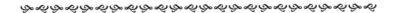

Foul play can also be involved. I had a case involving Dr. Albert, a scientist with no history of mental problems who reportedly committed hari-kari with a kitchen knife during an argument with his wife. He survived and was taken to a local hospital, where he was placed on life support. An investigation turned up evidence that for a period of a few weeks before the stabbing took place, this middle-aged man was engaging in unusual behavior. He neglected his hygiene and appearance. He was moody and began speaking in gibberish. Dr. Albert's wife insisted he had become upset about an experiment that was preempted at work. If supported by the facts, he could be considered a victim of job stress who became so despondent that he tried to take his life. His wife held power of attorney for medical decisions and opted to pull the plug — though he was in stable condition after being admitted to an ICU. Ultimately, the wife collected a sizeable death benefit.

Things are not always what they appear to be. No physical autopsy was performed on Dr. Albert. Poisoning by heavy metals, psychoactive drugs, or pharmaceuticals was never looked into by doctors. His body was cremated before any blood or tissue samples could be obtained. My suspicion, as a consulting psychiatrist to the employer's insurer, was thwarted by the destruction of the physical evidence. Without such information, too many questions went unanswered about why a man with no history of mental illness would decompensate in response to a not uncommon stressor and go on to inflict severe harm to his person. Psychological reactions tend to make sense, as do physical responses to life events. In this case, a simplistic conclusion involving job stress was advanced and accepted without a vigorous investigation of more nefarious possible explanations being allowed to take place.

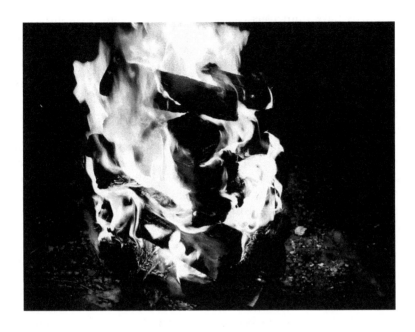

8 | Burn, Baby, Burn

Burn injuries not uncommonly result in some of the most complex industrial injury claims. Initial treatment provided through burn units at major medical centers can save lives. Often, a series of hospitalizations follows to perform skin grafting procedures and the removal of scar tissue. Pain control is crucial in the early stages of treatment, and with time, attention must be given to the potential of burn victims becoming dependent upon narcotics. Extensive burns can affect far more than skin, with there being a need to monitor respiratory and renal functions. Complex burn cases require a team of clinicians that can include plastic surgeons, trauma and orthopedic surgeons, infectious disease experts, pulmonologists, internists, pain management doctors, physical medicine consultants, highly trained nurses, and both physical and occupational therapists. Of course, any serious burn case will also result in the need for mental health services.

Burns have numerous causes. They include sun exposure, fires, chemicals, steam, molten metals, heated surfaces, frigid conditions, and other physical insults that damage the outer surface of the human body. Burns are classified as being first, second or third degree in severity with third degree burns being most serious. The extent of the burn area in a given individual is estimated as a percentage of total body surface. Hence, a third-degree burn affecting 40% of total body surface is extreme compared to a first-degree burn of 10% of body surface.

The California Labor Code governs how work-related injuries are administered. Since 2013, for an injured worker to receive permanent disability benefits for a psychiatric injury, beyond what that individual is due for any physical disability, the physical injury must be considered "catastrophic." Four examples of catastrophic injuries listed in the Labor Code include loss of a limb, paralysis, severe head injury, and severe burn injury. In a 2019 en banc decision, the Workers' Compensation Appeals Board found in favor of an injured firefighter by concluding that the nature of the injury, as opposed to the mechanism of injury, determines whether an injury should be considered catastrophic. In other words, both an injurious event and its aftermath must be considered. This is important because for many burn victims, a lengthy, painful course of treatment often follows the acute, horrible incident.

After stabilization of initial burn injuries, a victim can be expected to be dealing with a range of emotional and psychological challenges. Post-traumatic recollections of a fire or accident scene are often reported. Fear of death, disfigurement, and disability can come forth. As time passes, a burn victim's sensitivity to her appearance can manifest in an avoidance of public outings. Gratitude for survival and the care received can be intertwined with negative feelings of anger, despair and helplessness.

My role in the three cases that follow was to make clear that psychological injury can persist, as does the physical scarring left by being burned. Mental injury is all too real in instances of serious, permanent physical insult.

❧❧❧❧❧❧❧❧❧❧❧❧❧❧❧❧❧❧❧❧

Mr. Jones was a union welder employed by a construction company to repair heavy machinery. He was working on a leaking fuel tank on an earth mover when a spark ignited diesel fuel around him. The welder had performed the same type of repair work on many occasions, but apparently a safety measure malfunctioned this time. Recognizing his peril, the worker rolled on the ground in an attempt to extinguish the fire that had engulfed his protective clothing. A co-worker came to his aid and put out the flames with a fire extinguisher. His welding mask had provided some protection, but it was evident that emergency medical care was urgently needed. Mr. Jones lost consciousness while being flown by air ambulance to a trauma center equipped with a specialty burn unit. He spent the next three months hospitalized while medical care was provided for first and second degree burns covering 80% of his total body surface area. (Had the burns been second and third degree burns covering the majority of his body surface, survival would have been unlikely.)

We met almost a decade after Mr. Jones had been burned. In the interim, he had undergone more than forty surgical procedures. Many of the invasive procedures involved areas of the face, neck, arms, and legs. Complications developed around breakdown of skin tissue. He required reconstructive surgery of facial tissue, primarily affecting his nose. Chronic pain related to scarring and contractures was managed by two opiates he was prescribed. He also took medication for his disturbed sleep. By then, a 40-year-old married man, he had assumed the duties of managing his home. He had qualified for Social Security disability benefits, as he could not return to his welder duties and had significant physical limitations for other forms of work. His wife, whom he met after the accident, worked in the healthcare industry.

About a year after he was burned, Mr. Jones entered counseling with a psychologist. Psychotherapy continued for six years with a focus on post-traumatic images, feelings of depression, and low self-esteem associated with concerns about his appearance. During this time, he was also treated with an antidepressant for a few years, which he reported helped with sleep as well as anxiety while in public settings. Numerous physicians who had been involved in this man's case concurred that he was not up for the challenge of reentering the work force. Vocational assessment recognized his intellectual abilities yet emphasized his physical limitations, which made him a less-than-optimal candidate for most jobs.

In our meeting, I observed prominent scarring on Mr. Jones' face, neck, and extremities. He acknowledged being bothered by strangers staring at him but considered such behavior to be due to their ignorance. While life had changed because he was a burn victim, Mr. Jones saw himself as a survivor. My role was to describe his psychological response to a life-threatening and life-changing event. He no longer wanted to participate in counseling with a psychologist. I recommended to the insurer a trial of duloxetine, an antidepressant, approved by the U.S. Food and Drug Administration (FDA) for managing pain. If effective, his reliance upon narcotics might lessen. Ultimately, the judge considered the evidence and found this worker to be permanently and totally disabled.

In the case of Mr. French, I also evaluated a worker's ability to cope with the aftereffects of being severely burned. He was working as an iron worker when, on a hot day, sparks from a nearby construction site caught his clothing on fire. A fellow worker ripped off Mr. French's burning shirt. He was then taken to a university medical center where he was admitted to a burn unit for treatment of burns on his right arm, shoulder, and upper back. Approximately 12% of his body surface area was affected. Skin grafting took place using donor tissue from his lower extremities.

Mr. French described his recovery as physically painful. Return to duty as an iron worker was not recommended out of concern for exposure to the sun and the limited range of motion of his affected right arm. He requested access to a psychologist, whose records described Mr. French as dejected and troubled by memories of being burned compounded by his time in the hospital. While meeting with his psychologist, he came to accept that he should not return to his prior work, and a demand made by Mr. French's attorney led to retraining as a pharmacy technician. My report allowed the parties to settle this worker's claims with a recognition that he would continue to experience mild yet chronic post-traumatic symptoms affecting his mood, self-image, and interpersonal relations. His need for retraining, while justified given his permanent physical scarring, would result in a new career path that was amenable to the modest, yet persistent psychological difficulties.

In yet another case, I consulted with a roofer who had been burned on his dominant hand when hot tar spilled into a glove he was wearing. Mr. Garcia described experiencing excruciating pain while attempting to remove the glove, which trapped hot tar against his hand. His foreman took him to an area of the construction site where the roofer could put his hand into a bucket of cold water. He was taken to a local emergency room and from there was transported to a medical center with a burn unit. He came under the care of a hand surgeon.

A series of nine surgeries took place over the next several years to perform skin grafting and removal of scar tissue. Stabilizing hardware was inserted and later removed. Mr. Garcia had weaned himself off of pain medication following the last surgery. He saw a counselor who helped him to better accept his having been injured. Unfortunately, that outpatient treatment could not diminish his intense fear of potential injury if he were to return to roofing work. Again, my role was to make clear why this injured worker could not return to his former duties. Certainly, his physical injuries adversely affected his ability to take on the demands of roofing, but his persistent fears also put him at risk when working under conditions similar to those present when he had been burned. This 33-year-old former roofer would now need assistance in learning new skills for work within his restrictions. As a result of my report, an injured worker would have a future.

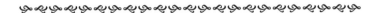

In each of these burn injury cases, we see how a single event at work can end an employee's chosen career. Burns, whether affecting a circumscribed area of the body or a more extensive region, often result in lengthy periods of treatment and rehabilitation. Along with multiple surgeries, there is often the need for mental health treatment, as took place in each of these cases. Just as physical scars remain, so will psychological symptoms. Disturbing memories, sensitivity about appearance, and diminished self-esteem should be expected. As with other serious health problems, such as cancer, burn victims become survivors whose lives are forever changed.

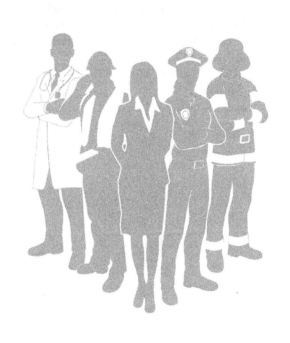

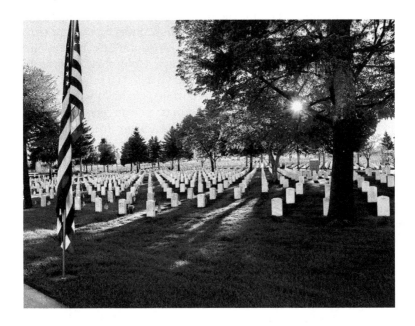

9 | 9/11

September 11, 2001, like December 7, 1941, is a day that
will live in infamy for America and humanity. I awoke that
morning next to my wife, with our radio alarm clock announcing
that an airplane had flown into one of the towers at the World
Trade Center. On the West Coast, it was still early on a day that would
prove to be increasingly horrific. Up and out of bed, we headed to the
kitchen for a cup of coffee, hoping there had been some mistake in the
broadcast. Instead, we spent time in front of a television watching a
second plane hit the adjoining tower. Then one of the towers collapsed,
followed by its twin. Having been in those structures on a prior visit
to New York City, it seemed impossible that we were watching mass

destruction of immense structures containing thousands of souls. It was all too real. Welcome to the 21st century version of war.

While this was not the first – nor the last – instance of terrorism on the U.S. mainland, it remains the most universally disturbing event for modern day Americans. As a country we now understand what citizens throughout the world have experienced. Terrorist attacks have occurred in Munich, Paris, London, Tokyo, Chechnya, Columbia, Nigeria, Iran, Brussels, and many other locales. They have involved schools, subways, sports events, places of worship, restaurants, nightclubs, and government embassies. Bombings, mass shootings, poison gas, fires, kidnappings, rape, forced conscription, and enslavement are tactics used to spread fear. While terrorism often occurs on land, it can also involve travel on the seas and aboard airliners.

September 11, 2001 led to wars in Afghanistan and Iraq. Security concerns have forever changed travel and commerce. While sparking individual and collective resilience, the event also aroused fear, mistrust, and post-traumatic distress. Nations still engage in war, yet entities of a different sort can also produce terror and large-scale destruction. Religious zealots, cults, gangs, and political extremists have demonstrated the will and capacity to disrupt daily life in free societies.

Not long after the towers fell in New York City, while on a business trip, I took time to visit a firehouse in midtown Manhattan that had lost eight firefighters to the structural collapses. Those who survived were working double shifts as fires, accidents, and medical emergencies had to be covered by first responders. The outpouring of support from the public was impressive. Like others, I went to the firehouse to say "Thanks." I also wanted to get a better idea of how these first responders were coping. The firefighters and paramedics I spoke to that day were grateful yet taxed, physically and emotionally. In the years that have passed, the toll of toxic exposure on those who were involved in search and rescue, as well as in cleanup efforts, at ground zero has become apparent. Chronic respiratory illness and immune system disease have resulted in an increased incidence of disability claims. Depression and post-traumatic stress have resulted in the need for mental health treatment and early retirement of workers who dealt with the aftermath from our nation's greatest terrorist attack.

War and terrorist events teach us that humans have evolved to a point where we do not react merely with acute distress followed by chronic illness; there are also opportunities for courage and selfless action. (Post-traumatic stress disorder came to the forefront during the Vietnam War. The same unhealthy response to acts of violence had been recognized in times past as "soldier's heart" during the Civil War, shell shock in World War I and battle fatigue in WW II.) Recognition of pathologic reactions to overwhelming terror has resulted in research into clinical treatments for victims of violence. Medicine, psychiatry, and psychology have developed pharmacotherapy, talking therapies, and adjunctive interventions to help survivors place disturbing events into the context of their lives.

Earlier in this book we considered the concept that surviving a life-threatening occurrence can strengthen one's mettle. (Recall the account of Ben, the battalion chief, in Chapter Six.) Recent studies of combat veterans have looked at resilience and post-traumatic growth as positive responses to horror. Not everyone reacts to terror by developing PTSD, just as not all exposed to the COVID-19 virus contract the disease. While disturbing dreams, intrusive recollections, avoidant behavior, and hypervigilance are commonly reported by military combatants, they also might experience a renewed appreciation for life. Those exposed to violent acts may initially respond with startle and panic. But beyond the acute event, they might also feel relief and improved confidence. First responders involved in critical incidents might succumb to burnout. Alternatively, such individuals may reconsider the importance of career versus other elements of their existence. This can lead to spending more time with friends and family as opposed to volunteering for overtime shifts. Hobbies can help to balance against work-related stress. Relationships can become more satisfying and supportive as a response to death and mayhem. While doctors typically are focused on diagnosis and treatment, much of human behavior is adaptive, even while surviving the worst of natural and man-made disasters.

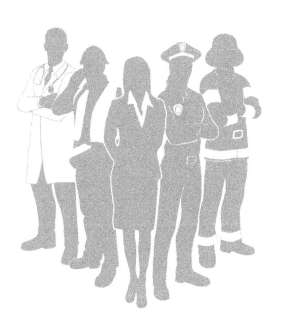

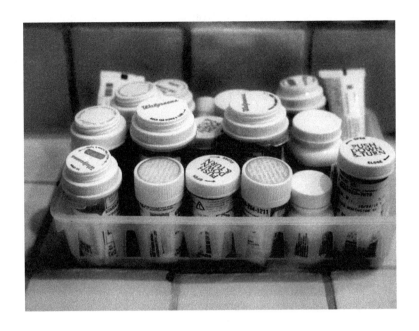

10 | Better Living Through Chemistry: Really?

Mr. Smith, a man in his mid-60s, sat across the desk from me, trying his best to disguise his distorted face. Like many employees seen in our offices, he had injured his back while engaged in work-related lifting activities. Pain medication, anti-inflammatory drugs, anticonvulsants, physical therapy, and injections had not provided sufficient relief from his chronic low back pain. Ultimately, he agreed to undergo an elective laminectomy to the affected area of his lumbar spine. His surgery was uneventful yet his pain was difficult to manage in the immediate postoperative period. Despite treatment with narcotics and sleep medication, Mr. Smith could not achieve enough pain relief to experience a restful night's sleep. Then one of his doctors introduced a new drug at bedtime.

Olanzapine, a psychotropic drug for treatment of schizophrenia, taken at a low dosage when needed, allowed the patient to relax and finally to enter a state of peaceful sedation. It felt miraculous to Mr. Smith. Unfortunately, when discharged from the hospital, he didn't notice that olanzapine, a psychiatric drug, was not among the prescriptions he was provided.

On his first night home, Mr. Smith was miserable because his pain once again prevented him from falling asleep. He took the provided medication as directed. He applied an ice pack as recommended. Still, his first week recuperating was marked by daytime discomfort and un-relenting pain at night. At his initial follow-up appointment with the spine surgeon, Mr. Smith was informed that the surgical results were as expected. The wound was healing properly. The patient acknowl-edged that he no longer had that annoying numbness in his right leg. He implored his surgeon for more of the drug that had helped him get to sleep. Instead, the surgeon prescribed a sedative. It didn't work. Mr. Smith became so desperate that he consulted with his long-time family practitioner, who provided him with a one-month supply of olanzapine. It worked! Blissful, heavenly sleep every night that Mr. Smith took the drug! When he didn't take it, the nagging pain led to tossing and turn-ing, which resulted in his wife sleeping in their guest room. At a return visit, his general practitioner assured him that the wonder drug was not addictive and wrote a second prescription with several refills to follow. When consulting with the surgeon, Mr. Smith neglected to inform that physician about his continued use of the "sleep" medication.

With sutures removed, physical therapy moved forward. Mr. Smith did not experience complete relief of his low back pain, but the improvement was noticeable. He was able to reduce his reliance upon the narcotics taken for pain. The surgeon scheduled the next checkup in two months. Mr. Smith's demeanor brightened. He and his wife planned to take a trip to his family's homeland in Europe because he could not return to work at the grocery store. His use of olanzapine at bedtime continued, now prescribed by a new doctor who took over the practice for Mr. Smith's trusted GP. No one mentioned potential side effects to the patient, who knew only that it provided continued restful sleep that he could count on.

Nine months after surgery, the spine surgeon reported that Mr. Smith was fully recovered from the invasive procedure. Even though he had residual limitations involving lifting and other strenuous activi-ties, he was pleased with the outcome. He was getting by with over-the-counter medication for his low level, nagging discomfort. He expected to retire with a small pension from his many years as a member of the grocery clerks' union. A disability examination was scheduled with a re-spected neurologist whose opinions would allow his claims of a work-re-lated lifting injury to be settled. Mr. Smith continued to take the wonder drug night after night, week after week, month after month. Life seemed good again. He and his wife were contemplating a cruise to celebrate his retirement.

At the evaluation with the neurologist, Mr. Smith was asked about his use of olanzapine. He took offense when the evaluator asked about any personal history of psychiatric treatment. Why would the doctor want to know if someone with a back injury had been hearing voices or having unusual thoughts? The neurologist recommended to Mr. Smith and his spouse that he discontinue the use of the drug because of the potential for permanent side effects involving involuntary muscle activity. The patient didn't recall ever previously being told there might be such a risk. Nevertheless, he complied with the recommendation, and it soon became obvious there was a big problem. Its name was tardive dyskinesia, known in the medical community as TD.

TD is a frightening movement disorder brought on by the use of antipsychotic medication. It is typically seen in the population of chronically mentally ill who have taken psychiatric drugs to address auditory hallucinations and other psychotic symptoms such as delusions. The drugs work by blocking nerve endings in the brain. These medications are powerful agents that can stop patients from hearing the voice of the devil or end grandiose fantasies. Yet as the dosage increases or the duration of drug use persists, the risk of developing side effects goes up. Perhaps most troubling is that the side effects can be permanent, and there is no cure. Mr. Smith was now forced to get by without the medication that had brought on desired sleep and that had ended much of the disruption of his daily life. His daytime existence was colored by uncontrollable movements in his face that involved lip smacking, a protruding tongue, and grimacing, which caused others to see him as disturbed or "crazy." He became depressed, angry, and frustrated. Life would never be the same. How could this happen? He didn't deserve this.

Remember that Mr. Smith's primary health problem had been back pain, which improved as a result of surgery. However, this man now had a permanent, involuntary movement disorder for which there was no cure. The movement disorder was an unintended but foreseeable consequence of wanting relief from insomnia in his immediate postoperative period. The sedating medication was actually an antipsychotic used for an "off label" purpose. Not uncommonly, prescription drugs are instituted to address symptoms for which they were not approved by the Food and Drug Administration. For example, certain blood pressure medicines, known as beta blockers, have been found to reduce shakiness or tremors. Those drugs are then routinely used to help patients with those types of nerve problems who don't necessarily have hypertension. The difference between antihypertensives and the antipsychotics is that the antihypertensives aren't associated with the possibility of serious side effects. Consumers need to trust their doctors yet be their own advocate. Advocacy requires asking about potential risks and deciding if they outweigh the reward. The "cure" can be worse than the illness. That is the take-home message in the case of Mr. Smith. There was no happy ending.

ഔ-ഔ-ഔ-ഔ-ഔ-ഔ-ഔ-ഔ-ഔ-ഔ-ഔ-ഔ

A 2018 study published in the Journal of the American Medical Association found that 59% of adult Americans take at least one prescription drug and that 15% take five or more drugs. Essentially, three of every five people in our country routinely take medication. These startling statistics have consequences. In recent years, there has been understandable concern for the overuse of antibiotics which can result in potential resistance by microbes. The opioid epidemic is real, and physicians have been asked to more closely monitor their patients' use of these powerful, yet potentially addicting, pain killers. At the same time, another epidemic rages uncontrolled – obesity. Not surprisingly, many of the most commonly prescribed drugs are for treatment of hypertension, heart failure, diabetes, high cholesterol, and gastric reflux, each of which can contribute to weight problems.

These chronic health problems are directly associated with a society that has seen its citizens become lethargic and obese. When I was a medical student some four decades ago, my colleagues and I were taught that there were basically two forms of diabetes, type 1 and type 2. Type 1 diabetes is a hereditary illness seen in children. We were taught that type 2 diabetes was associated with lifestyle and became expressed later in life, with it being commonly known as "adult onset" diabetes. In 21st century America, we now see type 2 diabetes in 8, 10, and 12 year old children. Does anybody think the solution is one or more of the latest pharmaceutical wonders? There is no magic pill for the problem of obesity. The answer is not more medication but rather diet, exercise, and teaching healthy habits to young people and their parents. Otherwise, we will see a continued rise in disability, chronic illness, and death occurring earlier in life than we have seen for many decades.

We psychiatrists also use drugs to treat common yet complex problems of living. We are not immune from the influence of the drug companies that market their wares through us and directly to the public. Among the most widely prescribed medicines are the antidepressants. Many people experience depression and other mood disorders, such as bipolar disorder, at some point in their lives and are treated with pharmaceuticals. Some of the most commonly prescribed psychotropic drugs, those used to treat mental disorders, include the antidepressants sertraline, bupropion, and fluoxetine. (Generic drug names are used here for medications more commonly known to the public by their trade names.) The anti-anxiety agent alprazolam is popular as well.

Some antidepressants, such as duloxetine and trazodone, are frequently used for complaints of chronic pain and insomnia. The antipsychotic drugs aripiprazole and the extended-release form of quetiapine are among the most profitable drugs prescribed by all physicians. The sleep agent zolpidem is regularly prescribed by doctors of all medical specialties. The anticonvulsant gabapentin developed to treat seizures is now used to reduce chronic pain and as a mood stabilizer. The concept of better living through chemistry has become well established in medicine and psychiatry.

It turns out that while psychiatrists are uniquely trained to write prescriptions for antidepressants, anti-anxiety drugs, sleep agents, mood stabilizers, and antipsychotic medications, most patients treated with these types of psychotropics never consult with a psychiatrist. The use of antidepressants has become so commonplace that the majority of Americans taking an antidepressant are under the care of a primary care physician, a nurse practitioner, or some other non-psychiatric clinician. In many cases, no specific psychiatric diagnosis is listed in the patient's chart. The antidepressants do not typically have the serious side effects seen in the case of Mr. Smith, yet they can cause other side effects, such as sexual performance problems and weight gain. Some individuals experience withdrawal-like symptoms when discontinuing the use of an antidepressant. Prescription medication for insomnia and anxiety problems can lead to tolerance and addiction. So, there is no such thing as a free lunch when it comes to chemical answers to dealing with loss, fear, pain, and sleeplessness.

Not all psychiatrists share my view that psychiatric drugs should be used only when necessary and not usually indefinitely. These drugs should best be viewed, I believe, as a component of treatment that includes counseling or psychotherapy directed at the behavioral problem or dynamic issues in each unique individual's situation. Even in other areas of medicine, there are limits to what can be expected from taking a drug to address chronic illness such as high blood pressure, elevated serum cholesterol, diabetes, impotence, and gastric reflux. Effective treatment almost invariably includes attention to diet, exercise, tobacco and alcohol use, along with other lifestyle issues. We'd all like it to be simple and take no effort. Too bad. It's time for our society to encourage individuals to take personal responsibility.

Just as there are warning signs of obesity in America's youth, there are also disturbing concerns about an uptick in mental problems in kids today. Depression, attention deficit disorder, autism, and bipolar disorder are being found at significant levels in our children. Adolescents are being diagnosed with personality disorders and drug addiction at alarming rates. Ultimately, the solution is not a cocktail of psychiatric drugs personalized for each minor. Our kids need structure and love that no pill can provide. The solutions to physical and mental disorders among America's children will involve more than drugs.

In my opinion, Americans as a whole have become more reliant upon and comfortable with the routine use of prescription drugs to address chronic health problems. This is not to say that medication, in conjunction with the body's immune system, is not effective in bringing about cures and remissions. Antibiotics for acute infections and chemotherapy for certain cancers can result in miraculous outcomes. Those situations are very different from patients becoming accustomed to taking numerous pharmaceuticals as though they were vitamins, supplements, or candy. It is not uncommon for me to consult on a middle-aged person's case and find out through my investigation of the records and a clinical interview that the patient is taking more than a dozen drugs prescribed by multiple clinicians for a panoply of conditions, often in the absence of coordinated care. Essentially, no one is in charge or managing things. The result is a person who is no longer in control of one's own health. Many of us pay more attention to what we put into the machines we operate than we do to the foods, chemicals, and drugs that we consume. Think about it.

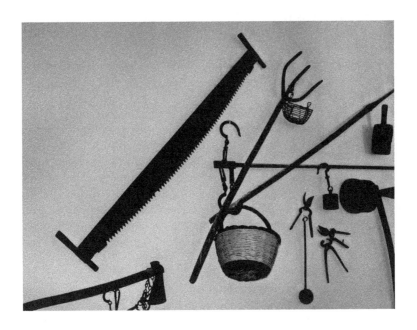

11 | We Call You the 'Hammer'

Even before medical students begin their clinical years of training, they learn an oft-repeated message: "See one, do one, teach one." Today's trainee becomes tomorrow's trainer. At Northwestern University, we were expected to practice venipuncture on a fellow student. Lucky for me, my pal Mark had actually been employed drawing blood at a hospital. He on the other hand was subjected to my anxious efforts at learning how to pierce the skin, find the vein, and withdraw the body's vital fluid. It's safe to say Mark was tormented by my early efforts, that too often produced more pain than blood. Thankfully, I did get better with time and patience on his part. Russians have a saying that applies here: "Repetition is the mother of learning."

We are asked as young students to function as instructors to our fellow pupils. We recite passages from literary works and give an interpretation. We practice scenes for school plays together. Most everyone recalls giving a book report in front of the entire English class and somehow surviving. My nerd friends and I really took delight in developing science projects to show off some concept such as gravity, wind resistance, or water tension! You could usually tell which kids would join the debate team in high school because they'd volunteer an answer to a question about sentence structure and then go off on some tangential discussion with the teacher. Members of the debate team often ended up attending law school and seemed to continue their penchant for arguing over stuff.

My first paid teaching position came while I was an undergraduate at the University of Colorado. While other sophomores were spending their free time at the gym or trying to impress their fraternity brothers, I had a work-study job in Dr. Goldstein's laboratory. By mastering lab cleanup and prep work, I developed a high skill level with biologic specimens. As a result, I was hired as a teaching assistant for a class in which I helped students examine tissue samples and microorganisms using light microscopes in lab-like settings. My role was to substitute for the professor and graduate students, who had more important teaching and research to accomplish. I saw myself as being of service to others while feeling valued by real scientists such as Dr. Porter and Dr. Wise. The work honed my skills and paid my rent. I also enjoyed it more than working in a restaurant or on a loading dock.

After completing my B.A. requirements early because I ran out of money, I interviewed at med schools and worked at the University of Miami with my mentor, Dr. Wise. That period of time exploring cell structure and South Florida was followed by my working in a lab in Boston, where I was fortunate to have funding for exploring the surface structure of the inner ears of guinea pigs. No major scientific breakthroughs came about as a result of my work in Miami or at Boston University. But I became proficient as an electron microscopist and lab assistant, which led to my working with biologists at Northwestern University Medical School (NUMS) while I began my medical studies. Microbiology was a required course for first-year med students at NUMS, and I was again hired as a teaching assistant working with my peers. I then set teaching aside for some years while I concentrated on medicine and psychiatry.

After finishing medical school, an internship, residency training, and a two-year fellowship, I was asked to teach forensic psychiatry to third-year residents in psychiatry at UCSF. The esteemed Dr. Diamond was no longer available to give his seminar entitled "Mental Health Law." So, I developed and implemented a new course that didn't use just one instructor. Instead, for the next decade, I made use of psychiatrists

50

and attorneys in an eight-week class called "Psychiatry and the Law." Subjects included ethics, civil detention, criminal responsibility, disability law, family law, sworn testimony, precedent legal cases, and the role of the expert witness. No trainee was expected to be a medicolegal expert after this introductory course, though they did gain a greater understanding of forensic psychiatry. Some trainees subsequently went on to obtain forensic fellowship training, which has influenced their careers.

One learns in life that institutions are not always benevolent. My course was eventually eliminated by a committee I served on that was tasked with making changes to residency training at UCSF. Not long after, I was asked to teach in the newly created forensic psychiatry fellowship. Over the next dozen years, I instructed trainees in the evaluation of individuals with claims of psychiatric injury related to work and other civil matters. No longer would I be teaching in a classroom but rather in the offices of my medical group, the Center for Occupational Psychiatry, on Market Street in San Francisco.

The forensic psychiatric fellowship at UCSF lasts one year and follows completion of medical school and a four-year residency in psychiatry. Completing the fellowship allows one to take the board certification examination in forensic psychiatry. (Completion of a four-year psychiatric residency is required for the board certification process in the overall field of general psychiatry.) The forensic fellowship at UCSF involves assignments at San Quentin State Prison, through the county court system, accessing sex offenders, and in family court. At the Center for Occupational Psychiatry, I oversaw fellows completing evaluations of individuals with claims for work-related injury, long-term disability, disability retirement, fitness-for-duty issues, and civil matters involving employment law.

The UCSF forensic psychiatry program is one of about four dozen accredited forensic psychiatry fellowships located at major medical centers around the United States. There are about a half dozen instructors at various Bay Area clinical and institutional settings. Only two fellows are selected in San Francisco each year. The fellows are in their late 20s or early 30s and hail from a variety of cultural and academic backgrounds. They typically have impressive resumes. Most want to learn about the legal system with the prospect of broadening their career opportunities after completing the program. Some need a firm hand.

ఇ౾ఒ౾ఒ౾ఒ౾ఒ౾ఒ౾ఒ౾ఒ౾ఒ౾ఒ౾ఒ

Toward the end of my time as a professor teaching forensics, I had an unexpected experience with a particular trainee. Let's call this forensic fellow Dr. Frank. Like me, he was the son of an immigrant, so I thought he'd identify with the working class. That did not turn out to be the case. He resisted taking an assignment from a state system responsible for making determinations on the compensability of workers' compensation claims. The assigned case involved a young woman working as a retail clerk who was robbed at gunpoint and then fired by her employer for giving the robber the money in the cash drawer. Dr. Frank apparently had better things to do than complete the requested evaluation. He really wasn't interested in the clerk or anything I might teach him.

The evaluation went forward after I made it clear to program representatives that the claimant would have the right to file a complaint with licensing authorities about Dr. Frank's conduct. I promised to join the claimant in any such complaint if he continued to refuse to cooperate. After Dr. Frank's interview of the claimant, it was apparent he was not a willing participant. Despite having all the necessary correspondence and records, Dr. Frank delayed getting the draft of his report to me for review purposes. His work product was seriously deficient and needed substantial revision. I learned that this trainee had blocked my emails, wanted to file a complaint of abuse about my teaching style, and had no intention of completing the report.

As his professor, I had suggested that Dr. Frank take a writing class. That suggestion was considered "abusive" because he had graduated from an Ivy League college. Additional allegations of abuse stemmed from my stating that a medical student with far less training would have been expected to do a better job than he had demonstrated. Dr. Frank completed the task only after our department sided with the claimant. Nevertheless, my supervisee wished to go forward with his complaint to the university about my teaching. However, when he learned that I had his emails from the past year, which demonstrated a pattern of disinterest and disrespect for the people we serve, the doctor no longer wished to proceed with a formal complaint process. The assignment was completed. The robbery victim could now receive appropriate benefits. However, the initial response of the department had been to side with the trainee over the interests of the claimant. I was left with some doubt about the university's commitment to high quality education, rigorous standards for its students, and service to the community.

Dr. Frank was not the only trainee who resisted my critical feedback. These are professional students who are used to success and accolades. Grade creep is a real phenomenon in America. It starts with high school students benefitting from taking honors and advanced placement courses. Essentially, a good grade in those classes results in the student getting extra credit that translates into an artificially high grade-point average. The ambitious pupils and their parents come to know how to game the system.

At the university level, the instructors are in turn evaluated by their students. While well intended, this assessment of educators leads to professors wanting to be liked by their trainees. As is common at medical schools, the students at UCSF are asked to rate each teacher's effectiveness. To be promoted or to receive desired tenure, professors are evaluated based upon productivity in research, grant funding, ingenuity and patents, leadership and administration, curriculum development and implementation, and teaching assignments. Consequently, many professors become chummy with undergraduate and graduate students for whom they have responsibility to teach and assess. The end result is a "you scratch my back and I'll scratch yours" educational system.

UCSF is an institution of higher learning dedicated solely to the health sciences, with schools of medicine, nursing, dentistry, and pharmacology. Research conducted at UCSF either directly involves patients through clinical trials and double-blind studies or is laboratory based yet potentially applicable in shaping treatment protocols. The university uses a qualitative grading system, with students rated outstanding, excellent, good, needs improvement, and failing. This translates into letter grades of A+, A, B, D, and F. Note that there is no grade of "average," equivalent to a "C." While evaluating trainees as their professor, I had no way to describe a student as average. This system contributes to grade creep and a sense of entitlement.

Over the years, I had many trainees who were highly motivated and serious about improving their skill set. There were also some I considered to be spoiled children. Those individuals did not easily accept constructive feedback, much less critical review of their work. Not everyone deserves a good grade or a superior assessment of their progress. Some young doctors cannot see themselves as undeserving of praise. The goal should be to produce competent professionals, not prima donnas.

❧❧❧❧❧❧❧❧❧❧❧❧❧❧❧❧❧❧❧❧

While some UCSF fellows complained like Dr. Frank, most took the study of psychiatry and the law as a serious endeavor. One such individual was Dr. O'Brien. He was the son of a renowned physician and researcher. He had attended a number of prestigious universities. He and I ended up in a verbal confrontation that made both of us uncomfortable. Another forensic fellow had let me know that I had been given a nickname by more than one group of fellows. It wasn't Dr. Bob. I was told, "We call you the Hammer." Upon being apprised of this descriptor, I responded, "I've been called worse things." Frankly, my parents would have been proud that their son was considered by his students as some type of professorial enforcer.

Early in his one-year fellowship, Dr. O'Brien and I met in my office to review his progress. He had been assigned three cases to evaluate in our offices, in addition to his duties at other sites, such as the state prison. The conversation was just between the two of us.

Dr. Bob:	"This is the third time we've met to discuss your written work product and my recommendation to you is the same. Take more time, and get me something you'd be proud of."
Dr. O:	"It's a draft."
Dr. Bob:	"Well I don't care what you call it. I'd prefer a report that didn't require me to take five hours to edit. I'd prefer one that didn't expect me to be an English teacher. I'd prefer that you'd get me a document that was not filled with misspelled words, incomplete sentences, and run-on paragraphs. Then we'd be able to focus on your case formulation and the pertinent medicolegal principles that should be addressed before the final report leaves this office with my signing off on it."
Dr. O:	"I told you, it's a draft."
Dr. Bob:	"You're not hearing me. You can call it an 'Ishkabibal' for all I care. I don't want it. I'm not here to function as a proof-reader for you. I expect someone with your level of training to produce a written account describing a person who is in some fashion interesting. You need to get me a story that is like a novella or a newspaper column. OK? If you do your job, then I will help you on quality control so the report can assist others in administering to the claimant's case."
Dr. O:	"For the third time, it's a draft."
Dr. Bob:	"All right. Since you've brought up the number three, I will again remind you that this is the third time we've met to discuss your work product, which has been inadequate. I'm a great fan of baseball, and in my assessment, you've had three strikes. You don't get to give me another 'draft'. You're out."
Dr. O:	"What are you saying?"
Dr. Bob:	"Good. Now you're listening. What I'm saying is that you will not get me another written mess with the expectation that I will fix basic grammar, sentence structure, and spelling. If that were to happen, I won't talk to you about it. I will instead call up the chairman of our department and tell him to kick you out of this fellowship. Our chair was my professor when I was at your stage of training, and I treated him with respect. I didn't argue with him when he instructed me to improve in a specific way. So, I will also ask him to contact the national boards and make sure you can never sit for the certification exam in psychiatry because you are arrogant and a potential menace to patients. That is what would happen if you were to provide me with a fourth 'draft'."
Dr. O:	"I understand."
Dr. Bob:	"Excellent. So, when we meet after your next assignment, we will be able to concentrate on the forensic issues related to a particular case and not be distracted."

I never had another problem with Dr. O'Brien. We both knew he could do the work expected of him. I learned from my office manager that he left our offices crying following the discussion about 'drafts'.

I recall thinking that was a hopeful response on his part. Teaching can be tough love. If you take it seriously, it's not for sissies.

Several years later, Dr. O'Brien approached me at a professional meeting. I was still a professor at UCSF, and he was a board-certified forensic psychiatrist.

Dr. O: "Dr. Larsen, how are you?"
Dr. Bob: "Good. And you?"
Dr. O: "I'm fine. Do you have a minute?"
Dr. Bob: "Sure. What's up?"
Dr. O: "Do you remember we had a discussion about my writing style some time ago."
Dr. Bob: "Yes." (While thinking, OK, here it comes.)
Dr. O: "No one ever did for me what you did. No one ever called me out on the quality of my work or my attitude. As a result of what and how you got through to me, I am now respected in my area of the medical community."
Dr. Bob: "You're welcome."

That was the last time the two of us talked. He died not long thereafter at an all-too-early age. But before he died, he taught me a valuable lesson. Be confident enough in your own value to accept deserved critical input from others. Reflect on what you can do to avoid repeating bad behavior. Show gratitude to those who help us to be better people.

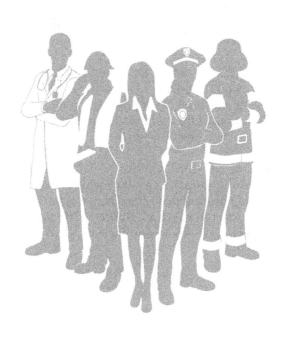

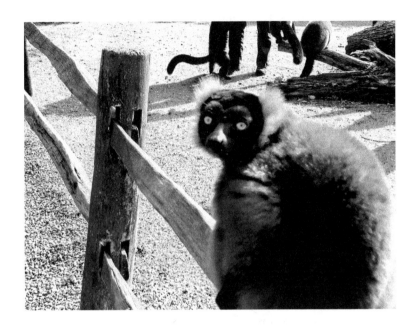

12 | Is He Believable?

As an instructor of doctors learning the role of a forensic psychiatrist, I have emphasized the importance of assisting others to answer a crucial question: "Can we believe the individual being evaluated?" Credibility is central to all opinions that follow that determination. This is true whether the case involves an alleged crime, a pending divorce, concerns of child endangerment, a civil tort, a disability claim, fitness-for-duty status, or some other legal/administrative proceeding. The parties' attorneys, the judge, the jury, the claims administrator, the employer, and the retirement board all need to know whether the individual telling the story can be believed, and to what degree.

Forensic psychiatrists and psychologists are utilized in a wide range of administrative and legal settings. The most salacious cases involve crimes of multiple murders, such as committed by Andrea Yates, or serial killers such as Ted Bundy and Jeffrey Dahmer. Those stories end up as front-page news and captivate us all, given the nature of the violent acts committed but also because of the character and mind-set of the perpetrator. Evaluations by mental health experts are conducted in the course of homicide investigations, as well as in trials to assist the trier of fact in making decisions about the accused's criminal responsibility, fitness to stand trial, ability to participate in one's defense, capacity to appreciate proposed sentencing, and other legal issues.

Criminal proceedings routinely use mental health experts to address legal matters. Frankly, while I have been involved in more than 10,000 cases over a period of more than three dozen years in which medicolegal issues were pertinent, I stay away from criminal proceedings like the plague. At a voyeuristic level, I find those sordid sagas fascinating, as do many of my fellow citizens. But I'd rather not get up close and personal to people who commit violence upon others, no matter what their psychological makeup might be. The same holds for pedophiles. Those folks are not merely dangerous to children, but they can also represent a threat to adults.

I do though have great respect for my colleagues who function as expert witnesses in criminal cases where mental issues are of major concern. As a member of the American Academy of Psychiatry and the Law for many years, I have attended numerous presentations by psychiatrists, psychologists, and legal experts on topics relevant to criminal cases. I have had the good fortune to get to know some of the most highly regarded experts in the subspecialty of psychiatry that addresses gruesome crimes. I have great respect for the doctors who render opinions so courts can adjudicate matters involving murder, rape, molestation, and other acts of violence. It's just not my cup of tea.

If one practices long enough as a psychiatrist, one hears some very unusual tales. Aside from scenarios of suicidal depression, paranoid delusions, paralyzing anxiety, and closed-head trauma, there are stories that involve implausible accounts that do not easily conform to typical forms of mental illness. As an occupational psychiatrist dealing with a broad range of claims of physical injury, emotional distress, and interpersonal conflict, I am frequently confronted with sagas involving exaggeration of symptoms, report inconsistency, overuse of the healthcare system, and outright misrepresentation. Although these difficult cases do not represent most folks seen for psychiatric assessment, they are neither rare nor obvious to discern.

Symptom exaggeration can occur purposely and with conscious intent to deceive. Doctors refer to persons who engage in that type of behavior as malingerers. Over-reporting symptoms and complaints can at times be seen in claims for physical injury involving the back, the neck, or the upper extremities. Subjective complaints related to those types of physical injuries can be extreme and unexpected, given the nature of a particular insult. In cases of symptom exaggeration, response to standard treatments is limited and recovery delayed. Similar scenarios are found in the fields of internal medicine, gynecology, neurology, gastroenterology, and every other area of medicine.

Embellished symptoms can include reports of dysfunction involving pain, sight, hearing, touch, and temperature. Motor function affecting walking, talking, gripping, and grasping can also seem excessively impaired. Nervous system problems including balance, coordination, vision, cognition, and even seizures are at times exaggerated. Psychological symptoms and complaints can also be excessive. Sometimes, out of frustration, a patient might report being suicidal just to be taken seriously by a primary care practitioner or an emergency room clerk.

Certainly, there are instances where the person reporting extreme or unusual symptoms is aware of doing so. In those cases, one is usually attempting to achieve a goal. That goal could involve time off from work, exemption from military service, a greater disability rating, designation as part of a protected class, or a number of other "rewards" for being found to be sick or infirm. People can also be unaware that their complaints are inconsistent with an illness based upon physiologic or anatomic abnormality. These patients are viewed as having psychosomatic problems. It turns out that much of what doctors treat as "stress" is really physical complaints produced by psychological distress.

Common conditions that might include a psychological component are migraines, gastric ulcers, skin rashes, erectile dysfunction, tremors in the extremities, and chronic pain. Less common forms of psychologically-based physical symptoms include tunnel blindness, pseudoseizures, and psychogenic paralysis. Historically, physicians considered these presentations to have a hysterical element and labeled them as "conversion disorders." Under contemporary nomenclature, these conditions have been designated as "somatoform disorders" or currently as "somatic symptom disorders." The physical complaints might not always have an anatomic basis but are real to the person who is suffering. It can be very difficult to treat such persons because they often resist accepting that some illusory psychic dynamic could be causing their physical distress.

When considering why a person's symptoms are exaggerated, attention must be given to the possibility of conscious malingering or lying, and of unconscious psychosomatic conditions. An additional category of mental illness, however, may account for a presentation of exaggerated physical or mental complaints. Munchausen syndrome was a descriptor used by doctors for some years to categorize persons with unusual presentations. The diagnosis harkened back to the fictional account of Baron von Munchausen, a German nobleman prone to spin tall, entertaining tales of his life. The current diagnosis is that of a factitious disorder. Such disorders are reserved for cases in which individuals feign, prolong, and self-inflict illness and injury.

Like the malingerer, an individual properly diagnosed with factitious disorder is aware of reporting extreme or unusual symptoms. The difference is that patients with factitious disorder volunteer for risky procedures that often create real damage. The malingerer knows better than to undergo unnecessary back surgery, while a person with a factitious illness looks forward to the procedure. Individuals with factitious disorders have been known to inject foreign substances into their body, to open surgical wounds, ingest hazardous chemicals, and take prescription medication at inadvisable dosages. It is hypothesized that persons with factitious disorder have the goal of remaining in the role of a patient, perhaps to receive attention and support. At times. this can prove to be very risky and even fatal.

Distinguishing between the diagnoses of psychosomatic illness, factitious disorder, and malingering can be tricky. All involve the reporting of symptoms and complaints that are excessive, unusual, or unexpected. A colleague of mine at UCSF studied cases that come up in clinical settings, such as in hospitals and outpatient clinics, as well as in forensic evaluations. Dr. Stu Eisendrath has found that the diagnosis in a given individual can fluctuate among all three forms of symptom exaggeration. Depending on the circumstances, the individual might or might not be aware of how one's actions and accounts might alter medical care and related benefits. Dr. Bob Wallerstein, chairman of the department during my psychiatric residency, told trainees, "The diagnosis can change from day to day." That is apparently the case for presentations of exaggerated symptoms, which makes arriving at an accurate diagnosis so difficult.

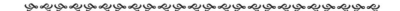

For example, take the case of Mr. Williams, who was a 60-year-old man when he was referred to my office by the judge assigned to his workers' compensation claims. By then, his injuries dated back almost one decade to a work-related motor vehicle accident. As a result of the accident, Mr. Williams underwent back surgery and extensive chiropractic care. He continued working for his employer as a salesperson for a few years after being injured though he made use of increasing amounts of medication to deal with his pain. With time, new complaints such as neck pain developed. A psychologist taught Mr. Williams relaxation techniques that reportedly helped to relieve his pain to a degree. However, it began to spread throughout his body even after he retired. Muscle cramping, fatigue, weakness, and falls followed. He began to use

60

a cane and then a wheelchair when venturing from home. He came to depend on numerous drugs to address complaints involving pain, sleep, mood, and daytime fatigue. Spinal injections brought temporary relief.

Mr. Williams became convinced that every one of his spinal vertebrae was defective. He saw himself at increased risk for developing total body pain as a result of his perceived genetic predisposition. His pain was reported to disappear during brief periods when he described himself as "paralyzed." He tended to seek out opinions from physicians with supposed expertise in managing cases of migratory, diffuse pain. He refused to settle his claims while making use of four different law firms over the years. He was also inclined to reject the cautious opinions of well-regarded clinicians.

As I combed through his records, I began to understand why the judge wanted Mr. Williams to undergo a psychiatric evaluation. Managing his medical and administrative issues was becoming increasingly complex and ineffective. In addition to my two-hour interview of Mr. Williams, I considered his psychological test results, consulted with the evaluating orthopedist assigned to the case, and gave careful attention to extensive medical records and deposition transcripts dating back almost three decades.

Mr. Williams had been repeatedly beaten by his alcoholic father throughout childhood. Interestingly, he did well academically and went on to work successfully in a number of sales positions. Coincidentally, his wife of many years was reported to also suffer from debilitating chronic pain. I learned that two of the couple's three children were deceased. One died in a car crash, and the other was killed by her remaining sibling, who was subsequently estranged from his parents. In addition to his primary complaint of pain, Mr. Williams was treated for urinary incontinence; memory problems; and neurologic difficulties, including intermittent paralysis.

During the interview, Mr. Williams was a bit irritable, and he became tearful when discussing the deaths of his children. He emphasized his physical complaints and made clear his anger at the insurer. The psychological testing was consistent with an individual of average intelligence who endorsed virtually every form of psychiatric illness. An orthopedic evaluation demonstrated a degree of disability in the areas of the neck and low back with no explanation for the claimant's diffuse pain, much less his reported paralysis. Videotape surveillance revealed he was far more functional than how he presented to clinicians. In fact, recordings of his activities showed him to be capable of strenuous activity.

A factitious disorder was diagnosed, with consideration having been given to malingering. Mr. Williams had become convinced that he and his wife were cripples. His treatment included the use of habit-forming medication and another drug with the potential for permanent side effects. He was described as presenting with features of somatization involving unfounded complaints of total body pain, memory loss, and pseudoparalysis based upon unconscious factors and conscious distortion. I recommended a simplification of his drug regimen and avoidance of any invasive procedures. Essentially, I was telling the judge that one could believe only some of this man's report and that he needed to be protected from his drive for self-punishment via unnecessary and ineffective treatment.

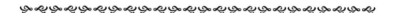

In cases where exaggerated symptoms and complaints are evident, my role is to help others involved in that person's case to better understand what underlies the production of excessive, unfounded difficulties. The malingerer's case should be dismissed. An individual with psychosomatic complaints might benefit from counseling and fewer diagnostic tests that tend to reinforce one's worst beliefs. The disturbed patient with a factitious disorder is best served by a healthcare system that does fewer interventions than demanded by that same individual who is intent on doing self-harm. Once again, we physicians must be guided in these cases by the directive of "Do No Harm."

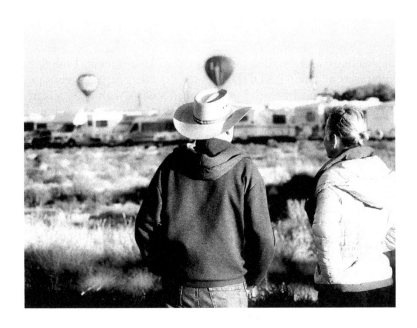

13 | Mentors Make a Difference

No one is a self-made man or woman. We are blessed if we grow up in a setting that encourages curiosity. We are blessed if we have parents, family, and neighbors who provide structure and security during our developmental years. Growing up a white kid in the Midwest during the 1950s and 1960s, I took much for granted. It may not have been an Ozzie and Harriett existence, but it was stable and nurturing. We always had a family home and decent food to eat, even if my mom overcooked the liver. Easter and Christmas were big events. Baseball gave us hope, excitement, and plenty of disappointment. While we had chores at home, we received an allowance for tasks completed. Good grades in school were rewarded as well, which was icing on the cake for Bob the Nerd.

I was fortunate to have many school teachers who functioned as parental surrogates. Miss Ginder, who taught second grade at Orland Park Elementary School, let me know I couldn't get away with bad behavior. She seemed ancient to me when she grabbed me by the arm and yanked me off the playground. All I had done was bite another kid as we were playing around. I suppose today I would have been sent to a child psychiatrist or psychologist for a clinical assessment. I might have been labeled as having ADHD, bipolar disorder, or the early signs of antisocial behavior. Instead, I got to spend a week with no recess in the company of my second-grade teacher, Mrs. Wile. I had a crush on her, and she probably felt more punished than me.

In third grade, I received the only "D" in my entire grammar school years. Orland Park had no kindergarten. I began first grade at age five because my mother was ready to let the public school system provide some discipline. No doubt she also wanted some relief from my antics. With a birthday in November, I typically was the youngest kid in my class. As such, I was often the shortest and quite immature. (Those characteristics became less endearing in high school.) Anyway, students were evaluated on "deportment," which is a subjective measure of behavior and obedience. Apparently, my incessant chatter during lesson time was a problem. Perhaps it was another sign of childhood psychopathology. In the late 1950s, it resulted in my receiving a "D" in deportment, along with mostly "A's" in real subjects. It also resulted in a stern scolding from my mom, though I don't remember my dad being too upset. Today, they might have started me on a trial of a psychostimulant such as Ritalin or placed me with a group of children considered to have a developmental disability. Somehow, I survived and didn't end up in prison.

Several years later, I again earned a "D" in school. I remember it well. All Carl Sandburg High School students were expected to take driver's education. I did not luck out when I was assigned the school's football coach as my instructor. He didn't much care for Humpty, the star in our school's version of Alice in Wonderland. When I almost drove a student-driver car into a ditch, the coach responded by coming close to eating his cigar while cursing at the same time. Despite getting high marks on the written exam, I ended up with a "D" for the course. The coach wasn't going to fail me because that might have led to us driving together again. Oh no! I was now my parents' responsibility. My mom didn't drive, and my dad had little interest in teaching me. Somehow, I learned enough to survive, though at times it made my passengers believe there must be a god.

Starting in the fifth grade, science, math, and foreign languages became rigorous. I took French, which went so-so. German was a better choice for me because I aspired to be a scientist. At that time, English, German, and Russian were the primary languages in the scientific community. That led to me studying Russian as well, in high school and college. Toward the end of grade school, the students who later ended up in honors classes in high school began to be separated from the pack based upon class performance and on yearly achievement tests. To me, tests were fun, like doing puzzles.

I still remember November 1963. My sixth-grade class listened as our teacher, Mrs. Anderson, informed us that something important had happened in our country. A television was wheeled in on a metal cart, and we watched as Walter Cronkite tearfully told the nation that our president had been assassinated. It was really scary and unsettling for us kids. Here was this father figure losing his composure on nationwide TV. My parents were Republicans yet were very upset by the president's death. My mom did not speak well of the Kennedys, but JFK did not deserve to be shot, for he was our president. Of course, this was when bipartisanship was a regularly utilized concept in the country's politics.

I had some fine teachers in grade school. Mr. Duncan, my fifth-grade teacher, was a tall, slender gentleman who always wore a suit. He also took no baloney from a bunch of boys who naturally wanted to emulate Huck Finn and Tom Sawyer. Fifth-grade girls are usually respectful and don't typically represent a problem to their instructors. Boys that age are wild things. Mr. Duncan used a ruler on us little rascals, and I don't recall any parent considering that to be abusive. He also had a habit of grabbing the worst offenders by their hair while pulling them away from their desks. We'd all snicker while the class disruptor, Mark, would get punished for his antics. I had not completely learned my lesson from the low grade in deportment for I too was selected by Mr. Duncan at times. However, I experienced a sense of glee when, try as he might, our teacher could not extract me from my seat by pulling on my hair. In those days, my mom used an electric razor to give my brother Guy and me our haircuts. There just wasn't enough hair to latch onto. That might have earned me an extra slap with the ruler, but it seemed worth the price.

While I was fortunate to have many good teachers in Grades 1 through 8, I don't consider any of them to have been mentors. It wasn't until high school that mentors entered my life. This is as it should be, I believe. Mentors are more than teachers. They are role models with whom there is the potential to have a mature relationship. Grammar school teachers were essentially daytime parents who taught us stuff while looking after us. An adolescent is capable of having discussions with an adult instructor where mutual respect can change the dynamic of the student-teacher relationship.

Beginning in the freshman year of high school, students were assigned to a home classroom. I was lucky to end up in Mr. Richard's biology class. For a kid interested in science, this turned out to be a gift. Mr. Richard probably considered himself to be a biologist and collector of animal specimens far more than a teacher. He was a massive person. Tall and heavy set, he lumbered when he walked. He was always proper and polite. He usually addressed us by our last names, such as "Miss Smith" or "Mr. Larsen." Our home room was located in a corner of the school, where it developed a reputation for the exhibits in the display case and the odors emanating from the classroom. We considered it normal to have aquariums containing fish, turtles, and snakes. On one school break, Mr. Richard ventured out to the southern part of Illinois and returned with an armadillo. That creature smelled pretty bad, and its waste products were beyond pungent. Hence, the well-deserved reputation of Mr. Richard's biological, experimental setting.

Some of us guys enjoyed staying after school to help out with the tasks required by Mr. Richard's animals, dead and alive. We became his brood. We learned how to maintain healthy environments for the live creatures while observing our instructor preserve those that had died. He had venomous reptiles and live black snakes that grew to 4 feet long. On one occasion, I was asked to retrieve something from the classroom's freezer. I must have jumped back at least 3 feet when I was confronted by two rattlesnakes. Each was in a perfect coil and very dead. Mr. Richard explained how he had preserved them by placing them in the freezer. Seemed reasonable.

Several months into our freshman year, Mr. Richard returned from spring break with three reptile eggs. The eggs were kept in an aquarium with a proper heat source so that the budding biologists could observe the snakes hatch and grow. These were no ordinary reptiles. Agkistrodon piscivorous is a venomous viper known for its ability to travel on land, up trees, and in swamp waters. The more common name for this poisonous snake is water moccasin. The babies were fascinating to observe. None of us students told our parents that we now had deadly, live snakes in our classroom. It was just part of the educational experience. We were becoming junior scientists! Then one day while feeding a baby snake with an eye dropper, the reptile bit Mr. Richard. Putting it back gently in its enclosure, our favorite biologist stated calmly, "Oh my, I've been bitten. Carry on class." Mr. Richard got himself to the school nurse and ended up hospitalized.

Our class learned that the biology teacher survived despite the bite wound becoming gangrenous. This development made Mr. Richard a folk hero to many students. The snakes were donated to the Brookfield Zoo, located in the Chicago suburb of the same name. Upon his return to our classroom, Mr. Richard exemplified the stance of the biologist we aspired to be by stating, "I always wanted to know if the antivenom would work for me." Our hero was allowed to finish up the academic year, but his contract was not renewed. I consider him a mentor because he presented us with a role model of more than a salaried teacher: an educator who encouraged his students to explore the world in search of life's mysteries.

Other mentors during those high school years were Mr. Tucker in chemistry and Mr. Potter, the band director. They reinforced my growing love of science, music, and experimentation. By the time I enrolled at the University of Colorado, I had a strong desire to study, learn, and absorb. I was a sponge for information. I did well academically by studying organic chemistry, calculus, and Russian. However, it was not until I got a work-study job in Dr. Lester Goldstein's lab that I began to truly learn about the scientific method.

Molecular, Cellular and Developmental Biology (MCDB) was a research institute at CU before it became a department that conferred degrees. Lucky once again, I took a part-time job as a lab assistant in Dr. Goldstein's lab, where the research focused on Amoeba proteus, a unicellular organism. I cleaned up after scientists, which included handling low level radioactive waste. Only once did I need to douse myself after dumping contaminated materials from above onto my person. With time, I became adept at fixing tissue with osmium tetroxide, using a diamond microtome to slice through cells mounted in epoxy resin, and separating proteins by gel electrophoresis. I was actually getting paid to participate in scientific studies!

During my tenure in Dr. Goldstein's lab, he likely published more letters to the editor of the New York Times than he did scientific papers. As a young man, he fought in Germany where he liberated a concentration camp of other Jews. He never talked to me about those experiences. He did instill in me diligence and attention to detail. He was appalled that I decided to pursue medicine instead of becoming a real scientist. He was correct when warning me that I would be trained to memorize in medical school when I could have been considering the mysteries of life. I owe Dr. Goldstein so much because he provided me with his honest viewpoint and never talked down to me. While strict, he was not mean-spirited in his oversight of a budding scientist.

While working in MCDB, other fine minds influenced me, such as Dr. Keith Porter and Dr. Larry Gold. Dr. Porter, who was our department chairman, provided me my first paid opportunity to teach laboratory techniques to fellow undergraduates. That bolstered my confidence and honed my basic skills as an instructor. Dr. Gold allowed me to come by his lab where the emphasis was on the study of viruses. While I was employed by Drs. Goldstein and Porter, Dr. Gold, then a junior faculty member who would go on to become known internationally for his research, spoke to me with the respect usually afforded a graduate student.

Lucking out once again, I was assigned to assist Dr. Gary Wise in Dr. Goldstein's lab. From early on, Dr. Wise treated me as a young protégé. One of the most wondrous experiences in my life was accompanying him into the electron microscopy suite. That day, we entered a world akin to landing on the moon when the magnification was turned up and we dove deeper into the cell's interior. Between graduating from CU and entering med school, I followed Dr. Wise and his young family to Miami where I again assisted him in his early career as a cell biologist and professor.

More than a mentor, Dr. Wise and his wife, Diann, have been good friends over the years. We have reconnected and stay in touch with mutual interests involving science, politics, and family. He has helped me to reestablish communications with Dr. Goldstein, who still teaches while in his 90s. Dr. Goldstein now encourages his former mentee in my efforts at submitting letters to the editor. It may no longer be the Vietnam War era, yet some issues in our society are worth debating. "Teach your children well."

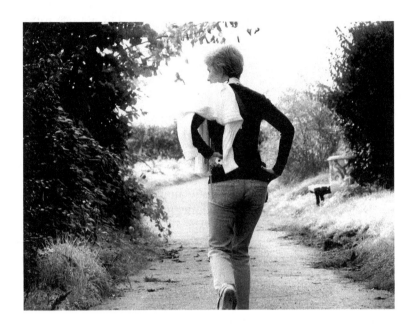

14 | Of Course, It's Personal

Ed was a veteran firefighter and paramedic. A man in his late 30s, he'd been doing the work for many years. Structural fires, motor vehicle accidents, grass and forest fires, medical emergencies, and disasters, whether natural or manmade, had come his way. Never had he made use of mental health services to cope with the loss, disappointment, and carnage. This time was different. This time it was personal.

Ed came to our offices upon referral from a local medical group that had a contract to provide clinical care to municipal employees suffering from work-related injuries. These cases usually involved acute low back strains related to lifting, whiplash symptoms after rear-end motor vehicle accidents, or respiratory complaints following exposure to noxious fumes. This case was not one of physical injury but was considered to be a "stress" claim.

Ed was on duty working a 24-hour shift when a call came in about a senior citizen who had collapsed at his residence. The address was well known to Ed because it corresponded to a property his father shared with several other men. A decision had to be made immediately whether Ed would take the call. His lieutenant agreed that Ed, his best paramedic, should go to the site. On the way, he hoped and prayed that his dad was not the subject of this call. Arriving on the scene, the team entered the residence, where they were taken to the victim who was lying on the floor in severe distress. It was his father.

Ed did not hesitate. He quickly assessed the situation. Ed's father was unconscious and had lost a lot of blood which was coming out of his mouth. His pulse was rapid, and he was struggling to breath. A fellow paramedic worked at putting an IV line in place. Ed was aware that his father was a regular drinker, and that meant this could be an acute hemorrhagic bleed. Along with liver damage and withdrawal seizures, heavy alcohol use can bring about esophageal varices. A certain type of hypertension associated with cirrhosis causes the veins in the lower portion of the esophagus to enlarge. The danger is that those veins become at risk to rupture under conditions where blood pressure remains elevated. Ed recognized his father's life was in a precarious state. He needed to be taken to an operating room immediately.

Commands were shouted out. The team was preparing to transport the victim. Ed was speaking to his dad to let him know what was going on, in the event that he might have some awareness. Then, with a convulsive coughing spasm of blood, the man who raised him became lifeless. The crew began CPR, to no avail. After what seemed like an eternity, the efforts to resuscitate were ended by a firefighter lieutenant at the scene. Ed's dad had died, and Ed was covered in his father's blood. Back at the firehouse, everyone knew Ed needed help.

It was obvious to the doctors at the occupational medical group that Ed required specialty care. A sprained ankle, they could address; but a grief reaction, compounded by the failed horrific attempt to save a family member's life, was way beyond their expertise. The medical group called my office for an urgent appointment. Ed arrived at our offices bereft. He had not slept much in the days since his father died. On leave from the firehouse, he busied himself with dealing with family and making arrangements for his father's funeral. His mother had died of cancer some time ago. Now both parents were gone. Nothing seemed to make much sense to this professional first responder who was used to dealing with life and death situations. This was different. This was very personal.

The diagnosis of an acute stress disorder was not difficult to make. We developed a plan to address symptoms involving disturbing emotions, intrusive memories, and fitful sleep. Ed and I met regularly for weeks. His department's managers and his fellow firefighters were concerned about his well-being. His family, including his siblings, cousins, wife, and children, shared in his grief. About a month into his treatment and leave of absence, a determination was made by the employer's insurer to deny Ed's industrial injury claim. His need for outpatient psychiatric care and a disability leave were considered to have been brought about by a non-industrial event, the father's death. Couldn't the death be viewed as a personal loss, while the failed effort to save his life be a legitimate employment stressor?

In discussing the claim's denial with my patient, he did not understand how the insurance company could be so cruel. Ed had been with his department for a dozen years and had never requested a leave of absence, despite having gone on many gruesome calls. He helped train new recruits. He worked collaboratively with management on labor issues. Now he was asking for help, and the answer was "You're on your own." No longer merely dealing with grief, guilt, and shame, Ed was pissed off. We agreed I would contact the claims examiner assigned to his case and see what could be worked out.

I called the insurer's representative and explained that my patient had been on duty, in uniform, and at the fatal call scene with the permission of his immediate supervisor. He had made a heroic effort to save a citizen's life, and the victim happened to be a family member. The examiner insisted it was personal and therefore not the responsibility of the city, the fire department or their insurance company. To which I responded, "Of course it's personal. So what?"

During a long process to resolve the coverage issue in Ed's case, an opinion was obtained from a non-treating psychiatrist hired by the insurer. That physician agreed that the condition was the result of employment. I cannot understand to this day why a competent attorney was not asked to review the claim. Perhaps some insurance personnel do not trust their own legal counsel. Ed considered getting his own attorney, but he opted to put that decision on hold after the insurer accepted his claim. He gradually improved with treatment. After some months, he was released, by me as his treating doctor, to return to work for his department where he was welcomed back.

The story unfortunately doesn't end there. Shortly after Ed returned to regular duty, a massive natural gas explosion rocked the city where Ed lived and worked. His firehouse responded to whole neighborhoods being blown up and burned to the ground. Ed tended to others in the community while concerned for his home and family. He recalled seeing an adult male running past him while literally on fire. Amazingly, some weeks after the gas explosion, Ed volunteered to plug an open gas line leak which in retrospect was extremely dangerous. This firefighter and paramedic kept doing his job, no matter what came his way.

Ed kept working at regular duties as a firefighter despite still having sleep problems and disturbing dreams. His treatment continued, though less frequently. He responded to more critical incidents involving serious injury and death. Finally, his claim was settled with the assistance of an attorney he had hired. The insurer agreed to provide future treatment as a means of supporting Ed's continued work, which was expected to expose him to more life and death situations.

The medical calls became more emotionally challenging for my firefighter as time went by. On further occasions, he recognized victims, some of whom didn't make it. Ed began second guessing his decisions about what treatment to institute. He ended up off work again, overwhelmed by the continued tragic nature of his job. Another claim was filed and accepted. Ed did OK when temporarily assigned alternative duties that dealt with safety inspections. He eventually returned to his role as a firefighter and paramedic, but it became increasingly clear that cumulative exposure to scenes of human misery had taken a toll. Now well into his 40s, Ed was burned out. He applied for and was granted a disability retirement, a decision he had struggled with for years.

Life has gone on for Ed and his family. His marriage remains intact, which is not a given for first responders suffering from PTSD. His kids are now young adults and doing well with their career choices. He has some contact with members of his department, but that is more a connection to the past than to his present life. Ed demonstrates resilience by training future paramedics. He has also adapted to life outside the department by owning small businesses. We still see each other periodically when he comes by to check in with his shrink. While facing his own demons, he has taught me much about the vulnerability and inherent strengths of being human and humane.

❧❧❧❧❧❧❧❧❧❧❧❧❧❧❧❧❧❧

Ed's case was complicated by the insurer for the fire department initially denying his claim. That decision complicated treatment and delayed provision of temporary disability benefits. Let us agree that insurance companies are not always our best friends. As long as we submit payments on time, they like us just fine. But filing a claim not uncommonly changes the relationship. This is not unique to workers' compensation carriers. Homeowner, automotive, health, and other insurers are usually not pleased when claims are submitted by an insured. Obscure policy clauses can negate coverage. If a claim is accepted, a premium increase might follow or eligibility for future coverage might end. Perhaps this somewhat jaded assessment is that of a physician who has dealt with numerous insurers over decades, but it is not mine alone. Once retired, I will not miss dealing with insurance coverage for workers who become patients for just doing their jobs. (The topic of insurance companies is central to cases portrayed in Chapter 30.)

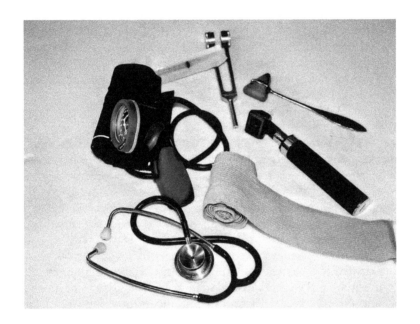

15 | Role Models in the Medical Arena

Relationships with the many role models who influenced my career did not end with the completion of my undergraduate studies. Additional role models influenced my career after I left Boulder. As a medical student with no family members employed as physicians, nurses, or health technicians, I had little understanding of what treating others required. Northwestern University Medical School (NUMS) emphasized memorizing human anatomy, such as the path of the pudendal nerve. My fellow students and I learned the signs and symptoms of infectious diseases, both the common and the rare. We were expected to understand how the body dealt with toxins and metabolized pharmaceuticals. By my second year at Northwestern, it was clear that Dr. Goldstein was correct. Unlike the curriculum in cell biology where students gave thought to how species adapt and evolve, my early medical education emphasized memorizing facts, pathways, and formulas. At times, the volume of information was overwhelming, and frequently it was neither interesting nor satisfying. I came to see that I could master the content of what was expected of a med student — but toward what goal? Time and an invaluable mentor would make that goal clear.

Training changes us. This is true of basic training for the military, the police academy for cadets, law school for aspiring attorneys, and certainly medical training for doctors. Medical students might start out a bit squeamish about exposure to blood and bodily fluids, but that soon passes. They then must become comfortable learning about the bad test results of a favorite patient. With time and experience, the med student develops a professional demeanor and the emotional distance that allows one to provide aid to others living with serious illness and injury. That change is a human process that requires young doctors to have not only a cache of facts, but more importantly, a capacity for empathy and understanding of another's plight. For those of us who had little prior contact with the healthcare system, we turned to our professors and clinical instructors to mold our character and to learn by their example.

In my second year of medical school, while studying infectious diseases and pharmacology, I found myself uncertain about what I might ultimately do with all of this knowledge. By then, I had heard lectures from physicians across a range of medical specialties. I started weighing my options. I really couldn't imagine becoming a pathologist, though my training in biology would have been very handy. My intuition told me I'd be better working with the living as opposed to conducting autopsies. Based upon my distaste for gross anatomy, it seemed that most surgical fields would not be a good fit. Although I could have become a technically proficient surgeon, it was a dirty type of work that didn't emphasize having a long-term doctor-patient relationship.

I had some idea about family medicine, because I grew up going to a general practitioner who cared for everyone in our family. From what I could tell, that doctor worked harder and longer than anyone, which wasn't that attractive. I had never been good at babysitting, which ruled out pediatrics. As much as I was attracted to the female anatomy, treating diseases of the urogenital system was not a pleasant prospect, eliminating gynecology. Ditto for urology and proctology. The field of internal medicine held some allure because it involved a lot of problem solving. That might work, and maybe my research interests could be incorporated. And then the field of Freud came into my consciousness.

Ironically, I never took a psychology class in college. The closest I came to studying human interchange and behavior as an undergrad was when taking two semesters of communications courses, which I found to be boring and mechanistic. Early in our medical school training, my class heard presentations from members of the psychiatry department. This caught my attention. Here were doctors trying to understand diseases of the mind and make sense of complex behavior. The part of me that enjoyed the challenge of chess found these concepts to be intellectually attractive. With little else to go by, I decided to make an appointment with the chairman of the psychiatry department, Dr. Visotsky.

The first time I walked into Dr. Visotsky's office, he welcomed me in, put his feet up on his desk, and lit a cigar. He was the chairman of the Department of Psychiatry at Northwestern. Dr. Visotsky had a good-sized office and a large desk on which he kept a large Rolodex containing hundreds of professional contacts. He referred to those contacts as his "floating crap game." I initially spent about an hour with this physician, administrator, and businessman. We were never interrupted and we had a delightful time. By the end of that first meeting, he had suggested that should I be serious about pursuing additional training in public health, I must look up Dr. Len Duhl at the University of California in Berkeley. I left with the impression that psychiatry had much to offer me, and a mentor was there if I wanted to avail myself of his wisdom and connections.

While others went off for spring break in our second year, I volunteered at an outpatient drug treatment program. I thought I knew something about drug abuse conceptually, but the patients in the program let me know how naïve I was. Something about intravenous drug use gives me the creeps. Moreover, anything that good, with all of its risks, is best to stay away from trying, even once. Often, it becomes far more than once. While working in the clinic, I developed great respect for the staff who got down with the addicts and helped them through recovery. That is, if the patient was motivated to change and stay clean. God Bless the Twelve Steps. Alcoholics Anonymous and its progeny give the alcoholic and addict, who have lost control, the structure, and support needed to resist the urge to once again drink and use drugs. In that adventure at the drug treatment clinic, I happened across a psych nurse named Janice, who became a girlfriend, role model, and mentor of sorts. She modeled a demeanor that was caring yet strict. She had the ability to call out patients who were exhibiting bad behavior while showing compassion for their pain. Not an easy task to assume.

One of the charismatic members of the psychiatry department at Northwestern was a professor named Francois Alouf. Dr. Alouf had a delightful French-Arabic accent and appeared to enjoy talking about taboo subjects like sex. He hosted a weekend workshop for students and faculty titled "Sexual Attitude Reassessment." Over that two-day seminar, lifestyle issues were openly discussed by homosexual couples, people in open marriages, folks committed to abstinence, and plain old straight heterosexuals. It all took place on the university's Chicago campus, where there was no chance of things getting out of control.

A men's group came about organically through the efforts of seminar participants spearheaded by a gay couple. So, what do you suppose a men's group in the 1970s did in Chicago? We got together at people's homes. We had pretty decent potluck dinners. There was a massage session that some found threatening but turned out to be relaxing, invigorating, and very safe. There was a bowling event to challenge our issues with sports and competition. All in all, this was pretty tame stuff for fellows dealing with what it means to be male. Thank you, Francois. You remain one of my favorite shrinks and mentors.

I knew that once I left Northwestern, I'd follow Horace Greeley's advice and go west. Before graduating from NUMS, I spent a couple of months at the University of New Mexico on an externship entitled Indian Mental Health. We made home visits to Native Americans, some of whom were being treated for psychosis, whether a correct diagnosis or not. Some of their homes had dirt floors and snakes that needed to be sent outdoors. I also had an externship at UCSF in the outpatient department, doing relatively little good for mankind while getting a delightful exposure to San Francisco. During this time, I was also applying to residency training programs.

Dr. Alouf's seminar on sexual lifestyles, combined with my participation in the men's group, resulted in my being rejected from my alma mater when applying to the University of Colorado's residency training program. I learned that the assessment of the most junior member of the faculty at CU was that I had an issue with my sexuality, a conclusion based solely upon my involvement in a weekend workshop and a men's group. Looking back on that odd experience, I'm pretty sure he was a closeted gay guy who thought I was pretty cute with my long hair and silver jewelry. The Indians I had spent time with in New Mexico also wore silver jewelry and their hair long, but why bother to explain? My mother had taught me that when people don't want you, just walk away. So, I accepted the assessment of the experts in Colorado that I was not a good fit for their program. Instead, I went to live in the City by the Bay. That's where I took Dr. Visotsky's recommendation to look up Dr. Duhl.

Although none of my peer group or the faculty at UCSF understood why a psychiatrist was interested in studying public health, I pursued a master's degree at Cal. I also found the time to meet my residency requirements at LPPI while moonlighting at multiple sites, including psychiatric emergency in Oakland. At Cal, I studied health planning from Dr. Heinrich Blum, who authored the notable textbook on the subject titled *Planning for Health*. In my last two years at Cal, I had another opportunity to study health policy through the Robert Wood Johnson Clinical Scholars program based at Stanford and UCSF. Done with my residency training, I learned more about how the healthcare field worked.

The Masters of Public Health program at Cal required a research and dissertation topic. Dr. Duhl was my faculty adviser. As mentioned earlier, he was a friend of Dr. Visotsky. Both were psychiatrists and academicians. Dr. Duhl had been assistant secretary of the U.S. Department of Health and Human Services in a Democratic administration. He was quite comfortable with having and expressing political views. I chose as my research subject the topic of impaired physicians. The individual stories were lurid. Yet the means by which licensing boards across the country deal with physicians who engage in drug and alcohol abuse, unethical behavior, financial improprieties, and fraud can be rather dry and institutional. Dr. Duhl was very different from most psychiatrists I interacted with in my clinical work. He was an educator, a health policy advocate, and a socialist. He was also a mentor who gave me permission to look not only at the welfare of the individual patient but also at the larger picture of the society in which doctor and patient live together.

While taking required courses and clinical rotations during my psychiatric residency at UCSF, I had time to do other things. Outside the program, I took classes through the Cal Extension campus in San Francisco on French and Chinese cooking. Within the residency program, trainees could also take elective seminars, and I took one from Dr. Bernard Diamond, one of the only American psychiatrists to be both a professor of psychiatry and the law. He was a psychoanalyst who became one of the country's preeminent forensic psychiatrists, publishing on the fallacy of the impartial expert witness, as well as on the unreliability of post-hypnotic testimony. He became attracted to the field of psychiatry when listening to radio broadcasts of the Leopold and Loeb trial as a youngster. He entered the field of psychiatry after World War II, when psychoanalysis was in its heyday. He was destined to end up as an expert witness in murder trials. He opposed the death penalty and always worked for the defense in criminal proceedings. His elective seminar, which lasted several months, was a must for me.

I was the only psychiatric resident to take Dr. Diamond's seminar that term. I was astounded that all of my classmates taking "Mental Health Law" were non-physician trainees. Apparently, psychologists and social workers saw value in learning relevant laws, while psychiatrists-in-training at UCSF did not. Dr. Diamond was a man of principle, and any disregard by the establishment did not bother him. He believed it was his duty to help a judge and jury to understand how a killer's psychopathology contributed to his actions and intent. Years later, when he no longer taught the seminar I had taken, our department needed a replacement course.

I came up with an eight-session seminar for third year psychiatric residents entitled "Psychiatry and the Law." The seminar made use of attorneys and psychiatrists familiar with areas of the law that relied upon the testimony of psychiatrists and psychologists. Dr. Diamond refused to participate because the time devoted to criminal law was insufficient, in his opinion. I recall him telling me, "Better that the trainees have nothing than pretend that one lecture can cover the topic." So, we disagreed, and the seminar took place without his participation. Dr. Diamond became my mentor as well as a model for ethical behavior. There was also the potential for me someday to be half the curmudgeon he was.

Another psychiatrist at LPPI, of UCSF, who influenced my career path was Dr. Carroll Brodsky. He was not only a psychiatrist, but also a physician trained in anthropology, who had written on topics related to disability and the culture of work. I crossed Dr. Brodsky's path while involved in my study of impaired physicians. He was a tall, handsome fellow who spoke deliberately. He could see I was interested in more than just treating neurotic patients and was generous of his time. I was becoming focused on how legal and administrative decisions were being made for individuals with mental problems. It may be that our politics overlapped or perhaps not. Dr. Brodsky encouraged me to begin taking cases of workers alleging work-related stress claims and helped me make connections to attorneys representing employees. Never once did he expect anything in return outside of serious collegial interchange. Ironically, over the years we ended up on opposite sides of cases being litigated, but there was always mutual respect for the positions taken. With his death, I miss his decency.

A major influence in my opting for a career as an occupational psychiatrist was yet another professor at UCSF. He was not a psychiatrist but instead a professor of occupational medicine. Dr. Joe LaDou was the chair of the Occupational and Environmental Medicine program at UCSF and welcomed a young doctor-in-training in the field of psychiatry. Dr. LaDou was probably an odd duck in the Department of Internal Medicine, just as I was among my psychiatric colleagues. We collaborated on producing three national seminars titled "Mental Health Issues in the Workplace." The conferences focused on a range of topics having to do with behavior, trauma, and culture in the modern work setting. I have contributed to Dr. LaDou's textbook published by Lange on the subject of occupational medicine. To this day, I continue to turn to him for advice. He is my colleague, mentor, and resource when it comes to issues affecting the welfare of working people and the institutions in which they toil. He is also my daughter's godfather.

Finally, when it comes to mentors, I must include a non-physician who has had a profound effect upon my professional path. Carl Brakensiek is an attorney who for many years was the primary lobbyist for occupational doctors and their patients in California. Previously, he worked for a state assemblyman. Many people have negative views of lobbyists, but they probably have not met Mr. Brakensiek. Aside from being a Dodger fan, I can find nothing to speak ill of him. He believes in the rights of workers. He is capable of compromise. He follows through on his commitments. We have known each other for more than three decades, and he has advised me in my various roles as an officer in a statewide medical society. I have been asked to testify before the California Legislature, and with Mr. Brakensiek's input, I didn't mess up. He has helped me to see how law and medicine come together in forming health policy that takes into account the principles of justice and welfare. For that, I remain grateful.

As a parting thought, I realize this attention to mentors in my life shows a relative absence of female role models. This is not to say that women haven't been peers, friends, and collaborators over time in my career. While I think of myself as having a strong anima, or feminine side, as Jungians see things, I might be mistaken. Raised in the mid- to late-20th century, I tended to turn to male teachers for advice and direction.

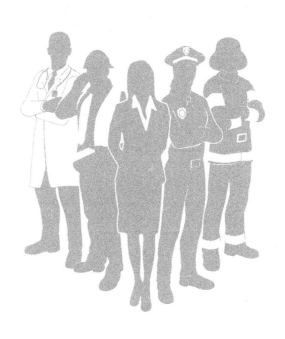

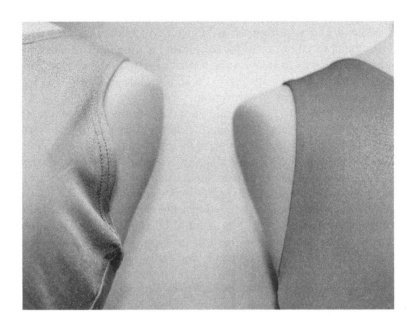

16 | Loss of a Limb

When we have our health, we take much for granted. Not everyone, though, is born with or lives out one's life with two healthy arms and two healthy legs. Some of us come into this world absent one or more fully functional extremities. The primary medical cause for surgical amputation is vascular deficiency associated with diabetes, a problem that affects mostly an older population. Cancer is another cause for doctors to remove a limb. In these situations, saving a life might require sacrificing an arm or a leg. For working men and women, physical trauma is the principal cause for the surgical amputation of a limb. In these cases, physicians must decide whether injured tissue is viable or not. Can the blood supply be established? Has gangrene set in? Have structural components such as muscle, bone, ligaments, tendons, and blood vessels been crushed, burned, or otherwise damaged beyond their capacity to be repaired? The loss of a limb under those circumstances is psychologically traumatic, especially in a person who has been healthy.

Most of us accept that we are mortal. We know that someday we will die, but probably not today. Similarly, a modicum of denial and avoidance allows us to take on risky activities that might cause injury. The government keeps statistics on the jobs and industries in which employees are at great risk of severe injury or even death. Logging, commercial fishing, roofing, and farming are consistently near the top of the list of employment sectors associated with a high risk of injury. Natural conditions, machinery, and human error contribute to the chances of a serious industrial injury. In this chapter, we hear the stories of workers whose lives were changed by an accident that took a limb. If you can, try to imagine what these trauma victims experienced physically and emotionally during the moments when they were crushed or mangled. Then consider how your life would be colored by multiple hospitalizations, surgeries, physical examinations and probing, clinical studies, scans, physical therapies, medication trials, and fittings for prosthetic devices.

❧❦❧❦❧❦❧❦❧❦❧❦❧❦❧❦❧❦❧❦❧❦❧

Jose was a teenager when he came to live with relatives in Central California. His early years were spent in a small town in Mexico where his parents had a farm on which they grew corn and raised livestock. As one of seven children, Jose was expected to work from an early age. He had just six years of public education when he began working as an unskilled laborer at construction sites in Mexico. After several years, he decided to head north, with his family wishing him well. Jose lived with his uncle's family while working as a ranch hand and in the fields picking crops. His job prospects were limited given his meager education and lack of English fluency. Still, the new job making tortillas at a local market felt like a step up for him. No more hot workdays in the sun, and he would receive an employee discount on all grocery items he purchased through his employer. With time he got more familiar with the tortilla-making machinery. He followed the instructions of his foreman without any debate. Six months into his employment, he had settled into a routine.

On the day Jose lost his hand, he recalls standing over a large industrial mixer, poring corn masa from a 10-pound bag. As he had done on other occasions, he stood atop plastic milk crates while he leaned over the stainless-steel machinery. When the crates gave way, he fell forward, dropping the sack of corn. He tried to brace himself with his right hand, which ended up in the churning mixture of corn, salt, and water. As he cried out, a co-worker hit the kill switch for the machinery. It took more than a half hour to free his hand from the metal whisks. A helicopter was summoned to transport him to a trauma center, where he learned that his dominant hand could not be saved. He had just turned 20.

During the initial hospitalization, Jose's hand was amputated. Additional surgery was needed to debride tissue from the stump that remained in the area of the wrist. After his hospital discharge, Jose was referred to an orthopedist who recommended the amputation be extended to just below the elbow. Some months went by before that surgery occurred. After the new stump had sufficiently healed, Jose consulted with a prosthetic expert recommended by his orthopedist. Not only was the initial prosthesis of little functional use, it did not even match the color of his skin. A second device was designed to use nerve endings to allow for some function of an artificial forearm and hand. It didn't work.

When I evaluated Jose, in connection with this injury claim, he had been dealing with his injury for three years. He complained, through an interpreter, of chronic pain at the stump where his arm had been amputated below the elbow. He also experienced a sensation of pins and needles that interrupted his sleep. While his hand was gone, he still experienced pain as though it was present, and he had learned that the phantom limb pain would likely persist. No further surgery was contemplated while steps were being taken to settle this young man's claims. As a result of my consult, Jose was referred to a Spanish-speaking psychologist to help him grieve his loss and to address the embarrassment he felt for his appearance. A trial of an antidepressant was instituted in an effort to lower his chronic pain. Most importantly, I recommended that Jose be referred to a university medical center with a state-of-the-art prosthetics department. Before his case was settled, he received an award for periodic revisions and updates of his prosthesis with the expectation that technical advances would improve the arm's function. Even with proper medical care, Jose's life was forever altered.

෴ ෴ ෴ ෴ ෴ ෴ ෴ ෴ ෴ ෴ ෴ ෴

In another case, a crush injury led to Jim, a logger, losing his leg. He was part of a team working in a forest in a far northern part of California, just below the Oregon border. He was operating a chainsaw while a co-worker used a tractor to push trees over. The crew had worked together many times. On this occasion, a tree that was being removed did not fall in the intended direction, and Jim was forced to run into the path of the bulldozer or have the tree come down on him. He ended up covered in soil with the blade of the bulldozer having landed on his right leg. He was extricated from the entanglement of the dirt and machinery, yet he lost consciousness before emergency personnel arrived.

After Jim regained consciousness in the hospital, he learned that he had lost his leg. A series of surgeries took place, ultimately leaving him with an above-the-knee amputation. The stump site required debridement of tissue, and the healing process went on for months following hospital discharge. Jim's response to his injury was anything but adaptive. He blamed the heavy equipment operator. He made heavy use of narcotic medication while it was prescribed. His use of alcohol increased. The doctor managing his chronic pain suggested he take an antidepressant. For a time, he snorted methamphetamine. Problems with the law came forth related to possession of illicit substances. Two years after he was injured, Jim entered a drug rehabilitation program that his doctor recommended, with the insurer covering the costs.

The good news in Jim's case was that he was still clean and sober when we met almost six years after he lost his leg. He was a regular at 12-step meetings. He had received outpatient counseling that had ended some time ago. He spoke in the most positive manner about the results of his consultation with the staff at the prosthetics department at UCSF Medical Center, whom he felt best understood his needs. A new titanium prosthesis equipped with an ankle shock had improved his function to the point that he could now go for a jog. On the other hand, his personal life, before and after the injury, had been tumultuous. He was not interested in further counseling and preferred to stick with going to Alcoholics Anonymous meetings. His permanent disability was so extensive he qualified for Social Security benefits. My role was to help the court to understand that, given this man's disposition, there was little likelihood he would now find value in additional mental health services or vocational retraining. Apart from his expected support through 12-step meetings, my psychiatric report emphasized the need for ongoing care to be provided for his prosthetic needs.

Jose's and Jim's cases share some common themes. Both workers were employed in jobs that involved the risk of physical injury. Both were injured as a result of coming into contact with machinery. Both lost a limb. Both experienced chronic pain. Both experienced feelings of depression that should have led to treatment. In each case, optimizing the prosthetic results was linked with how the injured worker would fair psychologically. While counseling and medication could be beneficial, assuring that the person had his function and appearance addressed through prosthetic treatment was probably more important. Jose and Jim needed to feel that they had futures and had not been forgotten. My role was to advocate for optimal medical and prosthetic care as beneficial to these amputees' well-being. Sometimes it takes an occupational psychiatrist to remind clinicians, attorneys, and administrators to treat the whole person. Assessing disability in cases of serious industrial injury is not enough.

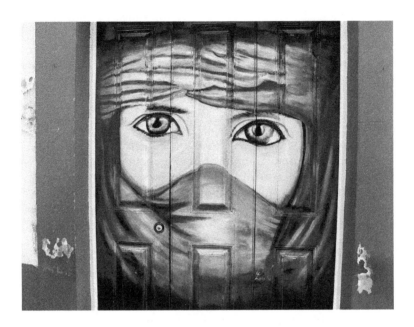

17 | I Am Unlovable

We met two years after Ms. Pham last worked in the laboratory of the food processing plant where she tested samples. This was her first job after obtaining her bachelor's degree from a major university. She had studied chemistry and food science, and as an immigrant from Vietnam, she was proud of her accomplishments. For six months, she monitored the quality of meat samples and of sanitation in the company's physical plant. As a woman in her mid-20s with a good job and benefits, her future was bright — until it wasn't.

Working alone in the plant's lab, this young scientist attempted to dislodge bits of meat tissue caught on the side of a meat grinder. She did so with great care while the machinery was in operation. Even so, her right hand was caught in the grinder. Immediately, she reached for the kill switch with her non-dominant hand, but it was too far away. No one was around. The machinery was powerful and began pulling her hand into its clutches. She screamed for help. After quickly removing a shoe, she extended her leg in an effort to contact the switch, but failed. The machine continued to slowly consume her arm. A food inspector heard her cries for help, burst through the doorway, and activated the switch, bringing the grinder to a halt. Ms. Pham passed out while co-workers extracted her mangled arm from the industrial-grade grinder.

When she awoke, she was in a hospital bed at San Francisco General Hospital, a trauma center. She felt pain in her injured hand and arm yet was unaware that the end of the affected extremity was gone. The record describes the injured hand as having incurred multiple fractures and having the appearance of ground beef. It could not be salvaged. She learned of her loss later in the initial hospitalization. What had been a healthy hand was now a memory, leaving her with a bandaged amputation stump in the area of the wrist. A surgical revision of the stump took place, and then she was discharged.

Outpatient treatment records documented Ms. Pham's healing wound. It was also apparent to her physical medicine specialist and a visiting nurse assigned to the case that she was not doing well emotionally. Even before she underwent another hospital stay for final surgery, she was in treatment with a psychologist. Symptoms of post-traumatic stress and depression were documented in the file. Months after the accident, Ms. Pham could not discuss what happened without screaming out. By the time we met, she had participated in hand therapy in an effort to train her in the use of her other hand. A prosthetic hand was manufactured. She dutifully attended appointments while giving every indication that she had given up.

Ms. Pham did not complain when filling out forms in our offices. The test results made clear that she was struggling with depression, anger, and anxiety. It seemed that her capacity to cope had been overwhelmed. I considered the potential need for hospitalization to stabilize her fragile state of mind. Despite her depression, she was well groomed and was exceedingly polite in her interactions with me. Yet throughout our meeting, she intermittently sobbed while averting her gaze. When asked how she would describe herself following the injury, she slowly articulated, "I am unlovable." My heart was broken.

This young woman had spent her early years in Vietnam following that country's civil war. She escaped during her teenage years and came to the United States with other family. Living in the Midwest, she learned English. After relocating to Northern California with her parents, she graduated from high school with honors. Following community college, she enrolled at a University of California campus, where she met her husband, who was completing his degree requirements. Correspondence from legal counsel gave me the impression that consideration was being given to closing out this woman's claims.

My report confirmed the diagnosis of a post-traumatic stress disorder. Additional counseling was recommended to address lingering sadness, fears, and embarrassment about her appearance. More importantly, I pointed out that the prosthesis that was in place was unacceptable because it had no functional value and resembled a cartoon appendage. I recommended that resolution of this employee's claims should not occur before there was a viable plan for retraining and workforce reentry.

Fifteen months went by before Ms. Pham and I met again. She had received additional counseling, but resisted taking any medication for her emotional difficulties. A consulting orthopedist agreed with my recommendation for a more functional prosthesis, and that process had been set in motion. Ms. Pham's mood was notably improved. She had given birth to a healthy baby girl, and her husband was about to graduate and begin a job search. She had looked into obtaining training as a pharmacist. She was receiving the benefits she needed and deserved. Follow-up psychological testing, while demonstrating emotional distress, no longer caused me to consider the need for inpatient care. The healing process had moved forward, and this formerly hopeless victim now had a future. Ms. Pham had adjusted to the lost limb, future treatment was guaranteed, and her disability claims were settled. My job was done. More importantly, no longer was she "unlovable."

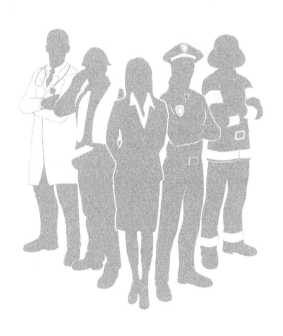

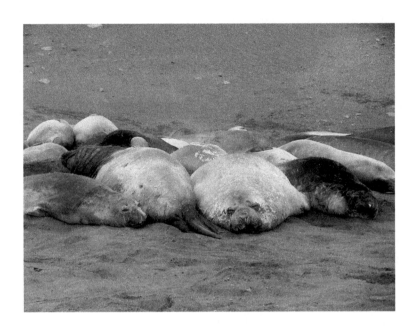

18 | Character: The Good, the Bad & the Ugly

"He's quite the character."
   "She's a Nervous Nelly."
   "Those twins not only look alike, but they act just like their mom."

"You can always tell a member of the Hatfield clan. They have that wicked temper."

"Her presence is infectious."

"He was a curmudgeon, even when on his best behavior."

"That girl is so thin-skinned. Compliments seem to irritate her."

"My supervisor is so competitive. Nothing's ever good enough."

Each of us has a personality and a unique character structure. People have different ways of coping or dealing with life events, big and small. Some folks are said to have a highly developed intuition, while many others lead their lives making mistakes of judgment repeatedly. What makes people interesting and complex is this stuff called traits, personality, style, and character.

Mental health professionals, while researching, diagnosing, and treating their fellow humans, categorize or label individuals based upon personal history, behavior, demeanor during interactions, and complaints that such persons put forth. Clinicians tend to broadly view patients with mental disorders as neurotic with manageable symptoms, psychotic or the severely mentally ill, and the characterologically disturbed. It should also be stated that being a bit different from others is not indicative of manifesting psychopathology or being screwed up. Vive la difference!

Since 1952, the American Psychiatric Association has taken responsibility for publishing The Diagnostic and Statistical Manual of Mental Disorders (DSM). This classification system is more limited in focus than the International Classification of Diseases, now in its 10th edition, which covers the entire field of medicine, including psychiatric illnesses. A fifth edition of the DSM has been available since 2013. DSM-5 replaced DSM-IV, which was published in 1994, replacing DSM-III and its forerunner, DSM-II. When I began med school, DSM-III served as the field's classification system during my training at Northwestern University and carrying on through my internship, residency, and fellowship years.

A major and somewhat controversial change contained within DSM-5 was a move away from a multi-axial diagnostic system. In DSM-IV, personality traits and the more pathologic categories of personality disorders were listed on a separate axis from other mental disorders, such as schizophrenia, mood disorders, and anxiety disorders. (For reasons that elude most of us, as of the fifth edition of the DSM, the abbreviated title no longer uses a Roman numeral.) Criteria were changed for a number of diagnoses. Inter-rater reliability or the likelihood that two doctors would agree upon the mental disorder diagnosis in a given patient has not improved. Some members of the mental health community have voiced concern about the influence of the pharmaceutical industry's support for study group participants who recommended certain changes. There was a rationale for these changes in making a diagnosis, yet some of us more rigid mental health practitioners were content with the system that existed. Change can be difficult for us all.

Whenever my nonpsychiatric colleagues mention how fluid mental disorder diagnoses seem to be, I remind them about conditions their patients have such as fibromyalgia, chronic fatigue syndrome, and complex regional pain syndrome. That being said, inter-rater reliability for diagnosing a personality disorder is low. Doctors will agree that a particular individual has maladaptive traits, yet there is likely disagreement about what those traits entail and whether they are of sufficient severity to result in a personality disorder being present. One person's borderline traits might be sufficient to be labeled as a personality disorder, depending on the physician or psychologist making the assessment. While it's not rocket science, the number of variables is infinite when trying to understand your fellow human.

The prior classification that I have used throughout my career utilized clusters to group together personality types having similar features. Cluster A included paranoid, schizoid, and schizotypal personality disorders. Cluster B included antisocial, borderline, histrionic, and narcissistic personality disorders. Cluster C grouped avoidant, dependent, and obsessive-compulsive personality disorders together. As this book is not intended to be a primer for the lay person on the subject of psychiatry, no attempt will be made to define these forms of "squishy" mental illnesses.

For me, the personality types contained within Cluster B are the most fascinating, frustrating, and terrifying to deal with as a clinician. They are no picnic for those whose family, friends, neighbors, and co-workers possess those characteristics either. In my humble opinion, they should best be considered the "Four Horsemen of the Apocalypse." In the unfortunate case that any one person has elements of the Cluster B personality types, such a disturbed individual could better be viewed as having been "Cluster F***ed." The prognosis in those instances is beyond horrible.

❦❧❦❧❦❧❦❧❦❧❦❧❦❧❦❧❦❧❦❧❦❧

Let us then consider a middle-aged guy named Dan who has been a businessman throughout his life. Dan's father was a successful real estate developer, and neither Dan nor his siblings wanted for material goods. They attended private schools and grew up in suburban comfort. If behavioral problems arose, the solution was to find a different school. No formal counseling, much less psychiatric services, were ever considered necessary by Dan's parents for any of their kids.

With financial help from his family, Dan tried his hand at various business ventures after finishing college. Some of these efforts resulted in bankruptcies, but Dan never saw himself as either at fault or having failed. He developed a reputation for cheating his business partners. He made a habit of filing lawsuits when outcomes of business arrangements didn't go his way. Dan bragged about his successes and lied about his failures. This included his personal life as well. He had been married and divorced multiple times. It was common knowledge in his community that Dan had been unfaithful with all of his wives. His anger was a weapon he directed toward those he considered to be his enemies and beneath him.

Dan has accumulated many adversaries over the years. While there were acquaintances in his life, he had no close friends. His sense of humor had the quality of a Don Rickles performance, where the jokes were always at the expense of others. Dan never reflected any laughter on his own foibles, as he had none, by his assessment. People who knew him were aware of his emotional volatility and also his tendency to be slighted by even mild criticism. This was a man who enjoyed humiliating others publicly, especially if they were at the center of one of his many grudges. Meeting with Dan was memorable in the same way that watching a cobra is enticing. Most people who were familiar with Dan tried to keep their distance.

Much more could be said about how Dan interacted with others. His pathologic lying, intense fury, selfish nature, and fragility are hallmarks of the Cluster B personality disorder tyrant. He had never been diagnosed with a psychiatric illness, such as major depression or bipolar disorder. He did not see himself as having flaws and certainly couldn't imagine reflecting upon his history of failed and conflict-ridden relationships. If he had ever entered outpatient psychotherapy, he would have represented a challenge to the most skilled clinician. Dan believed insight was overrated, and he saw no reason for him to change. While unhappy when he did not receive more recognition for who he was and what he had accomplished, he attributed those occurrences to the ignorance of others and their jealousy of him.

No medication currently existed to modify this man's behavior and attitude. Dan's self-assessment was that he was just fine. At that point in his life, there was little likelihood he would become a more tolerant or gracious person. He believed it was the world around him that should take lessons from his life. He had the equivalent of a terminal illness that prevented him from experiencing empathy, true joy, and intimacy.

Just because a doctor can make a diagnosis does not mean there must be an effective treatment. This is especially true when the potential patient lives a life of denial and self-adulation. The result is pathetic.

Fortunately, most folks weren't raised like Dan, who was led to believe he was special and better than those around him. Most of us make mistakes and at times suffer. Mistakes can become learning experiences that cause us to make adjustments. We might realize what brings about our suffering and thus avoid similar situations in the future. Upon reflection, we might start to see what responsibility is ours for the pain that has come forth. The wise elder with years of lessons learns, while the fool repeats practices that continue to bring on disappointment and futility.

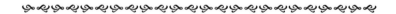

It should also be noted that idiosyncratic personality traits are not necessarily pathologic. A choreographer with a bit of hysterical flair might be a perfect match with the right ballet company. A touch of antisocial tendencies might make for a prolific car salesman who dupes customers while pleasing ownership. Most accountants, like professionals in general, do better with compulsive attention to detail. Few politicians survive without being somewhat self-centered or narcissistic. It is when personality and styles of coping become inflexible and excessive that interpersonal relationships become problematic. It is when a pattern of dysfunction becomes apparent that a personality disorder can be diagnosed. As with other lifestyle issues, everything is tolerated in moderation.

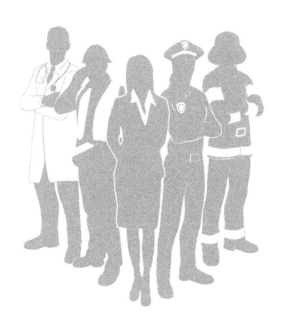

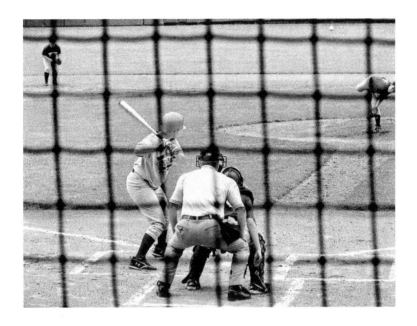

19 | The National Pastime

I **grew up a Cubs fan. I had no choice because my old man**
was a Cubs fan. I recall hearing of the great double play trio of
Tinkers to Evers to Chance, though I had no idea who those
ballplayers were or when they had played ball. During our
childhood and adolescence, my brother Guy and I watched the Cubs on
WGN or listened to the broadcast on a transistor radio. Jack Brickhouse
was the announcer, beloved by local listeners in the Chicago area. While
LA had Vin Scully, we had Jack. The Cubs battled the Cardinals every
year, usually with a dismal result. My dad could never get over his Cubs
having traded Lou Brock to the team that beat us year after year. The
Cubs played in one of America's great ballparks. Wrigley Field, with its
outfield walls covered in ivy, is a treasure.

Uncle Mike took Guy and me to our first game at Wrigley. We were unaware that Mom was having surgery that day so someone had to kid-sit. As we arrived on foot at the ballpark, I recall seeing men playing bocce ball outside the ballpark. It had the feel of an old city neighborhood with all the smells, sounds, and sensory input. Chicago Transit Association (CTA) buses buzzed by. Men were selling swag. Then we came upon that iconic entrance sign announcing, "WRIGLEY FIELD: HOME OF CHICAGO CUBS." Oh jeez, we had arrived. We had seats far from the action, but it didn't matter. We were in the cathedral of baseball. It was so ENORMOUS to a 9-year-old. The crowd was intense. You got to scream and yell as part of one gigantic hometown force. I don't recall the final score, but we stayed until the game was over. I was hooked.

I followed the Cubs through the remainder of my primary and secondary school education. During the summer months, we played ball in neighbors' yards and empty lots. Just bring a lawn mower and cut the weeds short. Balls lasted a whole summer. If someone hit one into the tall weeds, you'd search for it for as long as it took because you might not have a replacement. Bats were cherished. I had one bat that I loved. When I first got it, the bat seemed big and heavy. Like with clothes, you grow into a bat. One day in high school, I took it to PE class. I was the last kid picked for a team, but with that bat, I hit the longest shot of the day. Rather than running to home, I stopped at third and surveyed those other teens who seemed surprised that the fat kid had some power. The bat didn't survive the game as another guy broke it while batting. I took her home in two pieces. I drilled a hole and put in a wood screw to put the bat handle back together. I wrapped her with tape, but she was never the same.

It was years after my first visit to Wrigley that I returned. It was a pretty good distance from where we lived, and it cost money to go to a game. Listening on the radio or watching on television was free. Only one time in high school did I play hooky for a Cubs game, and it was worth it. A few of the guys planned to ditch school for a weekday game. All games at Wrigley were then played during the day, as the park had no lights. It was the only field in the majors at the time where games were called on account of darkness! The most notable happening of that game was Don Kessinger hitting an inside-the-park homer.

The inside-the-park home run is the most thrilling play in baseball. It involves more players, coaches, and umpires than anything else that occurs on a ball field. It also takes forever, and everyone in the park is cheering. Forget about a triple play or a grand slam. Nice, but no comparison. Kessinger was the Cubs shortstop and hit only 14 home runs in his 16-year career with the Cubs, the Cardinals, and the White Sox. Yet on that day, he thrilled the crowd with a shot to the outfield wall that allowed a tall skinny fellow to fly around the bases and score before the catcher had the ball. SAFE. It would be decades before I had the opportunity to witness Angel Pagan hit an inside-the-park homer at AT&T Park in San Francisco. It was a walk-off hit that ended the game in the 10th inning. The Giants were down by one run, with Brandon Crawford on second and one out, when Pagan launched one that sent us all home in a state of joy. It had been more than eight decades since the Giants ended a game with an inside-the-park home run. Got to love it.

In 1969, the Cubs were considered by many to be the best team in baseball. From game one until a time in September, they were the top team in the National League. Members of that team included future Hall of Famers Ernie Banks, Billy Williams, Ferguson Jenkins, Ron Santo, and their manager Leo "the Lip" Durocher. Durocher was a colorful character who took delight in three things at the park: winning, arguing with the umps, and getting thrown out of games. He had quite a wit and left us with memorable quotes. "Baseball is like church. Many attend, few understand." "Win any way as long as you can get away with it. Nice guys finish last." "I never questioned the integrity of umpires. Their eyesight, yes." It had been several decades since the Cubs had gone to, much less won, a World Series. Chicagoland was all behind the Northside gang. The team recorded a song "The Cubs Will Shine in '69." But they didn't. They died in September, giving up a 10-game lead to the Miracle Mets. I was crestfallen. I couldn't give my heart again, at least not anytime soon. It would be a decade before I'd watch a game again or root for a favorite team.

After moving to the Bay Area in the late 1970s, the pain of having supported the perennial disappointing Cubs had diminished enough that baseball reentered my life. During my residency training at UCSF, I attended several San Francisco Giants games at Candlestick Park. That was one chilly place to watch a game, especially at night. I met my kids' mother toward the end of my four-year residency, and we married two years later. We decided to leave San Francisco for the small community of Brisbane, located just south of the city, when we were expecting our first child. The Potrero Hill neighborhood where we were then living seemed a bit edgy; today it is considered quite hip. We could see the nightlights of Candlestick from our new home, and I began going to games. I became a season ticket holder, which required only a partial plan of 20 games. A big benefit was being able to upgrade to better seats when available.

My friend Richard and I went to a bunch of weekday day Giants games, especially when kids were in school. The crowds were smaller, and the seats were closer to the action. If you go to enough games, you'll see some stinkers. Boy, did we! One game stands out. Our seats were behind the visiting team's dugout. It was still the first inning, and the Reds were already up 5-0. I predicted, "The worst is over." Not so, as the final score ended up something like 18-7. It was an action-filled stinker, but the seats were fine, the weather pleasant, and the company delightful. I saw more games with Richard than anyone else because his schedule allowed for those workweek day games we both came to love.

Another perk for season ticket holders was the opportunity to purchase post-season tickets when your team had a good year. That happened for the Giants in 1987 and 1989. The World Series in 1989 was overshadowed by the Loma Prieta earthquake. That was the real tragedy, though my Giants being swept by the Oakland A's felt like the nail in the coffin for San Francisco fans. Owner Bob Lurie became frustrated with his inability to get a new facility for his Giants. The team came close to moving to Fort Lauderdale before a change in ownership took place.

Around that time, I was an officer in a medical association that wanted to put on a seminar during spring training. I floated the idea by Mr. Lurie, and he agreed to my proposal. "Optimum Performance in Professional Athletes" took place in Scottsdale, Arizona with the cooperation of the Giants management, coaches, and trainers. My colleagues and I gave medical lectures on relevant topics. We went to games and hung out at the resort where the team stayed. A good time was had by all.

It was also during the Lurie years that I wrote to Bud Selig, the acting commissioner of Major League Baseball and the owner of the Milwaukee Brewers. There had been some labor actions that had adversely affected the game, including one season that ended prematurely without any post season taking place. Fans were not happy. Mr. Selig responded to my letter by asking for my resume so that he could pass it on to the ownership committee in charge of selecting the next commissioner. I couldn't believe my luck. I had fantasies of closing down my psychiatric practice and flying to all the MLB ballparks to meet with owners and players.

The search firm involved was located on Park Avenue in New York City. I made a pact with myself that I wouldn't lie and that I'd be willing to take the job for half of the offered salary. I tried to ingratiate myself with the support staff of the search firm by bringing them See's Candies, a small bribe. My interview was short-lived when I advised against the concept of realignment, an idea promoted by some owners, including Mr. Selig. In my defense, that change to the game never came about. I now realize I was the ultimate dark horse candidate and never a serious contender. The fix was in with Bud Selig becoming the commissioner for the next two decades. Baseball was never going to hire an occupational psychiatrist to oversee the game, but they sure could use one at times.

In 1993, the Giants picked up Barry Bonds. He was a superstar who had grown up in the Bay Area where his father Bobby had played for the team. The new owners included Peter Magowan, formerly CEO for Safeway but at that time was dedicating himself to his team. That year, the Giants played at Candlestick, which was showing its age. The Giants had four All Star ballplayers in Bonds, Burkett, Beck. and Thompson.

The team won 103 games and lost out to the Braves, who won the National League pennant. Quite a year, as was 2000, when Pac Bell Park opened. It's now called Oracle Park and is worth a visit during the baseball season, whether one is a fan or not. It's a whimsical facility located on the Bay with spectacular views.

After 9/11, things changed in America. Airport security became more intense, for good reason. The nation prepared for war that came about, and I began bringing signs to ballgames. Some had to do with baseball. "He's a Cheater but He's Our Cheater." That one referred to the controversial Barry Bonds. Or, to goad the fans of the team in LA, "Dodger Dogs, Teeny Wieners. Hearts of SF, Giant Organs." There were also signs commenting on our times. They addressed the wars, vetoes of stem cell research, the recall of California's governor, and other matters of a political nature. Apparently, I offended a fellow season ticket holder who wanted me ejected from the park and arrested.

During the run-up to the 2004 presidential election, I was confronted by the head of ballpark security. He demanded that I hand over my signs and come down to Guest Relations or he would turn me over to a detail of three officers from the San Francisco Police Department (SFPD). "What if I don't like those options?" To which he responded, "So now you're gonna be a smart ass too?" After learning I was a season ticket holder who had purchased seat licenses, the security officer left me to confer with management. Meanwhile, I had a pleasant conversation with the officer in charge of the police detail who informed me that they liked my signs, but if the Giants considered me a nuisance, he would have to arrest me. He seemed surprised that my 18-year-old son was expected to register with Selective Service. We agreed that I would put the signs away for the time being.

Three weeks later, I helped to organize a protest at the ballpark over Memorial Day weekend. I had informed the Giants in advance. Fellow fans, including my friends Norm and Jan, arranged for placards and t-shirts reiterating what the sign had said. "IRAQ'S A MESS. BUSH AHEAD IN THE POLLS. WAKE UP, AMERICA." We consulted with the ACLU. FOX and NBC sent camera crews and reporters. Arrangements were made for a plane to fly over with a banner stating, "WAKE UP, AMERICA."

Guess what? The Giants changed their policy to allow political signs as long as they did not incite hate crimes, use profanity, or interfere with watching the ballgame. I took it a step farther by assuring there would be no misspelled words. The conservative fan who had complained still couldn't stand me, but many others enjoyed some of the more humorous signs, like, "Padres, the celibate athletes." In 2017, the country was getting used to our new president, and I again was approached by security. The sign that day read, "NEVER THOUGHT I'D MISS NIXON." We worked it out. Thank goodness for our First Amendment.

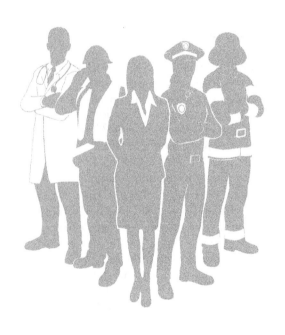

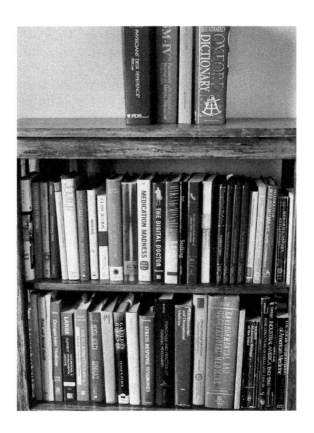

20 | Psychiatrists Are Also Real Doctors

It seems reasonable that surgeons, pediatricians, gynecologists, and family practice doctors are required to complete medical school. Why is it that to become a psychiatrist, one must also attend med school? Psychologists generally work with the same patient population, and their training does not require them to take classes in anatomy, physiology, and infectious disease. The reasons are multifaceted and important to understand.

Psychiatrists and psychologists diagnose, provide psychotherapy, or counseling, and engage in research on individuals with mental disorders. One key difference between these two professions involves the prescription of medication. Psychiatric medication, or psychotropic drugs, are used to treat symptoms of depression, anxiety, bipolar disorder, attention deficit disorder, schizophrenia, Tourette's syndrome, dementia, obsessive-compulsive disorder, and many other emotional and behavioral problems.

Psychotropic drugs are powerful. Antipsychotic drugs block neuroreceptor sites in the brain and have the goal of reducing hallucinations and delusions. Antidepressants act to boost the body's neurotransmitter chemicals, like serotonin. When effective, the desired response includes improved sleep, appetite, cognitive functioning, mood, and social functioning. Anti-anxiety drugs, or anxiolytics, attach to nerve receptors in areas of the brain associated with anxiety symptoms like phobias, obsessive thoughts, compulsive behavior, and nervousness. Mood stabilizers are prescribed to modulate swings from profound despair to manic elation in patients struggling with bipolar disorder. Psychostimulants are commonly a component of treatment for hyperactive kids. At the other end of the life cycle, drugs can help the elderly to deal with early signs of Alzheimer's.

For several good reasons these psychiatric drugs are used under the supervision of a medical doctor. The drugs can result in adverse effects that might require adjusting the dosage or substituting an alternative medication. Not uncommonly, patients being treated for mental illness have other health problems. Patients treated for cancer, cardiovascular illness, hormonal disorders, chronic pain, and neurologic disorders such as multiple sclerosis, often are also coping with depression and anxiety. Treating physicians must stay vigilant for the potential of drug interactions, including with medicine provided by another doctor. Additive effects can emerge when more than one drug is being taken, and effects become amplified. An example of such is consuming sleep medication after drinking alcohol. Similar additive effects can also result when taking multiple prescription drugs.

Taking a combination of psychotropics and medications for medical conditions can affect attention, balance and gait, judgment, and other bodily functions. A good psychiatrist is aware of the totality of the drug regimen the patient is using and of the patient's overall health issues. To avoid doing harm, there is often a need for a treating doctor of any specialty to obtain clinical laboratory assessment of kidney and liver functioning.

While there is a need for psychiatrists to be "real" doctors with basic medical training to prescribe drugs, there is a more central reason these doctors need to complete medical school. That reason is misdiagnosis. Any physician must consider that some other medical condition or the treatment for such is the basis for what, at first glance, looks like a standard case of major depression, psychotic illness, or generalized anxiety. Hypothyroidism mimics depression, and the proper treatment involves prescribing a thyroid hormone and not an antidepressant. Corticosteroids are used to treat many health problems, such as asthma, irritable bowel syndrome, and skin rashes. Those drugs are powerful and, in certain individuals, can bring on mania or psychosis. Symptoms of anxiety might be a reaction to life events or to caffeine intake, prescription psychostimulants, or recreational drug use. Just as a neurologist does not want to misdiagnose a brain tumor in a patient with the recent onset of headaches, so too a competent psychiatrist must "rule out" the possibility of a medical problem as the basis for what appears to be a primary mental problem. A case example will be used to bring the point home.

৯~৶৵৶৵৶৵৶৵৶৵৶৵৶৵৶৵৶৵৶৵৶৵৶

A few years ago, I was consulting on the case of Gene, a 64-year-old married man. Gene had worked for many years in construction, becoming a lead man overseeing a crew of skilled laborers. In the last year of his employment, he routinely became short-tempered with his crew. He voiced frustration with changes to the rules and protocols that had been part of his work at construction sites. When counseled by his manager, this long-term employee responded with an offensive and personal verbal attack. At that time, Gene was placed on a leave of absence by his employer. He then filed a stress claim and obtained legal counsel at the recommendation of his union representative. At the request of his attorney and the employer's workers' compensation insurer, Gene showed up at my office for a comprehensive psychiatric evaluation. The "injured worker" was accompanied by his wife of many years and an adult daughter.

Gene struggled with the standardized psychological testing he was asked to complete in our offices. His family was asked if they were aware of something that could explain his poor performance. They agreed that he was "stressed" and that it had been a long drive to our offices. The testing was interrupted as I opted to meet with Gene before expecting him to continue with test measures designed for persons with a basic academic skill set. There were few records to review in this case. Gene was a mildly overweight middle-aged man with no serious health problems. His only medication was a standard dose of an antihypertensive for high blood pressure, which was well controlled.

Gene insisted that his boss and fellow employees had been making his life difficult. He couldn't understand why so many changes were necessary for the crew to just do the job assigned. He had been thinking about taking an early retirement. His wife and his attorney had recommended that he discuss his options with his employer's human resources department, but he wasn't sure he could trust those people for good advice.

I detected there was something off about Gene's demeanor. He tended to hesitate before giving responses to what should have been

103

straightforward questions. I was left with the impression that some of what I was being told was made up. I interrupted the interview and, with his permission, brought Gene's wife and daughter into the meeting. It then became clear to me that Gene was confabulating, or filling in material that he could not recall. He had not had the breakfast that he reported having had to me. His family was protecting him from venturing out on his own, because he had gotten lost in their neighborhood recently. There were also instances where Gene made use of the wrong implement for a task. For example, he had been seen trying to rake his lawn with a broom. "Stress" again was cited as causing him to be confused.

I decided to perform a neuro-mental status examination developed at Stanford University. This is a series of tasks that takes a doctor about 30 minutes to administer. It assesses attention, immediate recall, short-term memory, simple calculation capacity, ability to name objects, judgment, decision making, and other cognitive functions. Gene's performance was impaired across the areas assessed, despite his making an honest effort. I gave the bad news to Gene and his family. He was not suffering from depression or a stress response. He was likely in the early stages of dementia. He needed to undergo a workup by his regular doctor, who would be able to identify more specifically what type of neuropsychiatric condition was present. With the correct diagnosis, a treatment plan could be developed. His family was devastated, while Gene seemed to be calm and not fully understanding my recommendation.

My report went out, and Gene received the recommended clinical measures that led to the diagnosis of Alzheimer's disease. A plan was made to assure his safety. He obtained appropriate benefits given his disability. His family came together in acknowledging that Gene had a progressive, dementing form of illness. There were no miracles.

Doctors, including psychiatrists, must search for the truth because it involves the health of their patients. I believe it is better to know what ails us than to pretend there is a nicer alternative. That's why psychiatrists need to be real doctors.

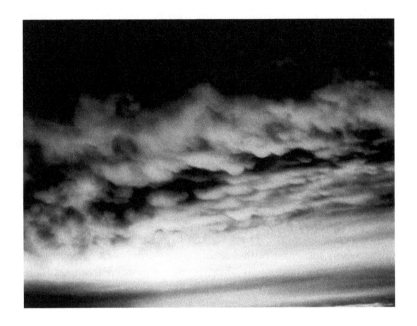

21 | Raped with a Gun

After reading through Janet's records, I found myself dreading the interview that would take place. There were emergency room records, medical records, a detailed police report, and a psychiatric report of a colleague hired by the employer's insurer. What do you say to a woman who has been raped with a gun?

The police report was unusually critical of the ownership of the convenience store where the assault took place. This was the third robbery in three months. The local police had made recommendations to improve safety measures after the first two. Those recommendations included improved lighting in the store's parking lot, installing a panic alarm, having a buzzer system to let customers in at night, and never having female employees work alone at night. None of the recommendations was implemented. The police report stated, "And now, we have a female employee who has been raped with a gun for two hours."

Janet was a 45-year-old woman who had worked for five months as a convenience store clerk in a semi-rural part of Northern California when a single male customer robbed her store. She had split up from her third husband around the time she took the job. She needed to support herself because she could not rely upon her estranged husband. Janet had been living in a studio apartment and had filed for divorce. She was getting by financially and was grateful for the assistance she had received from her church and a local food bank. Her children from a prior marriage were adults and independent of their mom. When she was offered an extra work shift, she took it, even if it meant working at night. She was aware that the store had recently been robbed twice, but no one had been hurt. So, she took the extra shift, which paid her time and a half. She could use the money to cover some of her legal expenses for the family law attorney.

It was a slow night. Janet recalled that it was getting near closing time when someone pulled into the parking lot in a pickup truck. She could see the driver was alone as he proceeded from the vehicle to the door. After entering and saying hello, the fellow headed for the refrigerated wall of beer. He selected a six-pack of a pricey craft brew and brought it to the counter. After seeming to reach for his wallet, the customer mentioned that he'd left it in his truck. He made it as far as the front door where he proceeded to turn the lock. She knew she was in trouble when he changed the sign to "CLOSED."

Back at the counter, the customer-turned-bad-guy pulled out a handgun and demanded all the cash in the register. The problem was that most of the money had been placed in a secure drop box, per procedure, one hour before closing. The robber was clearly furious when she handed over only about $80. She told him she had another $18 in her purse. He followed her into the store's back storage room where she kept her purse. Before she could remove the bills, he hit her on the side of her head, perhaps with the gun.

When she regained consciousness, Janet's hands were bound with duct tape that the robber had found in the storage room. Her head was throbbing as she lay on her back, staring up at the man, whose pants were around his ankles. She couldn't scream because the tape was over her mouth as well. As she felt the cold concrete against her bare legs, she realized things were about to get worse. Unable to keep an erection, the assailant cursed at her for wasting his time. He forcefully spread her legs and threatened to leave her dead if she resisted. Then she felt something cold and hard being shoved inside her. Terror overwhelmed her as she realized this monster was using the gun to assault her. It felt like an eternity before she passed out again.

Light was coming through a small window in the back room when the clerk heard her manager say, "Janet, what happened? Are you OK?" He pulled off the tape covering her mouth and binding her hands. The store manager handed her the pants she had worn to work and called 911. The police and an ambulance arrived within minutes. By then, it was morning, and her assailant was long gone. At the emergency room, Janet was helped into a hospital gown by a female nurse. Bruises in the areas of her scalp, wrists, inner thighs, and groin were photographed. Her vital signs were taken, and intravenous fluids were started. Another nurse took an account of the assault. After a time, a doctor examined her from head to toe. The exam was followed by a tetanus shot and an antibiotic administered through the IV.

A male detective asked the clerk to again recount her assault. She was aware that he was recording her statement. He gave her his card and indicated that he would be her contact with the department. Before being taken home to her apartment, Janet was given an appointment for outpatient follow up and told to use anti-inflammatory medication for the headache and aching pain throughout her body. Should the headache worsen, she needed to return to the hospital because she had been diagnosed with a concussion, though an MRI brain scan had shown no damage inside the skull.

We met six months later. Janet had not returned to work. She was receiving temporary disability benefits from her employer's workers' compensation insurer. Her assailant had not been apprehended. The outpatient care to monitor her injuries had been reduced to monthly visits at an occupational medicine clinic. Her doctor had been unsuccessful in obtaining authorization for a psychological consultation. Only after obtaining legal counsel had Janet found herself referred to my offices in San Francisco. That's where we met for our one and only encounter. Both of us were uncomfortable about my need to ask her to once again recount the night that changed her life.

"So, when this creep began to rape you with a gun, you must have known he was going to kill you. Yet, here you are, alive. Do you consider yourself lucky or unlucky?" She of course had no idea. Nothing any longer made sense. While her physical injuries had healed except for some lingering headaches, she struggled with fitful sleep, feelings of despair, anger at the rapist and the store owner, and frustration that she believed her situation was not being taken seriously. She avoided going by the location where she was assaulted, even if it meant adding five minutes to an outing. Unless it was necessary, she remained in her tiny apartment where she kept to herself. She resented having to meet with yet another male professional to answer questions about how "some sick motherf***er f***ed me with a gun."

I didn't ask Janet to tell me about all that took place that night in the convenience store. I asked her to tell me about her life as a kid, where she went to school, which family members she stayed in touch with, what went wrong in her marriages, and what other jobs she had held over the years. We also discussed the symptoms of anxiety, mistrust, and moodiness that now colored her existence. She indicated she would welcome having some counseling. She hoped I would not be offended if she preferred going to a woman. Though she had never made use of mental health care before the rape, she trusted her doctor, who said she should meet with a woman psychologist who had a good reputation in their community.

Janet had done some research on the Internet and learned that certain antidepressants might help "with this PTSD s*** that they say I have." We discussed the treatment options. I indicated that while it was unfortunate that nothing had been offered to date, it was not too late for her to benefit from outpatient care. She could be made more comfortable, and she would again have a future. However, I told her she should not trust any professional who might tell her she would come to forget what had happened.

For Janet to receive the help she deserved, I would need to be her advocate. If her employer had been negligent at having a female employee work alone at night at a location that had been recently robbed more than once, why would that same employer have selected a responsible insurer? The insurance company had also received a report from Dr. Williams, a psychiatrist, who took the position that in addition to her physical injuries, Janet had been subjected to emotional trauma. She would need some time to heal and probably could not be expected to return to work at the location where she had been assaulted. However, citing her three failed marriages, Dr. Williams had indicated that Janet's life was far from perfect, aside from the rape. Recommended treatment should have the limited goal of getting her back to her psychological baseline that predated the rape. Three sessions of individual psychotherapy were deemed to be sufficient by Dr. Williams!

I was already uncomfortable as a man explaining what it would be like for Janet to have been raped. I found myself outraged that my colleague had concluded that the injured worker deserved only three sessions to address the trauma. I eventually determined that I would have to make it graphically clear that my colleague had erred in his recommendation for this deserving worker to get what she needed.

In my report, I rebutted Dr. Williams' assessment by stating that no one could possibly know what Janet had gone through or might need to recover. That psychiatrist had made the case for Janet having had problems in her personal life that were not the insurer's responsibility. With that reasoning a limited course of treatment could be viewed as adequate. I suggested that Dr. Williams was likely healthier psychologically than Janet had been, though that is debatable. I went on to state that if, in a hypothetical construct, it was the psychiatrist who had been sodomized with a gun, he would probably want and need more than three sessions of treatment. Certainly, Janet would also need more than three sessions.

I made it apparent that I was not sure what the correct number of sessions should be, but I was certain it wasn't three. If the options were to authorize three sessions or none, I recommended that Janet be given nothing. At least that would be honest. Giving her three sessions with a psychologist would be akin to allowing a surgeon to perform back surgery but not close up the wound. After three sessions, Janet would be told treatment was over and that she was on her own. Better to give her the message that she had survived and no one cared.

Sometimes, we must be blunt to make a difference in people's lives. My report was admitted into evidence along with the report of Dr. Williams. At trial, the judge found in favor of Janet receiving outpatient mental health services for as long as the treating clinicians could justify, which turned out to be much more than three sessions. The judge had found my reasoning persuasive. Some months went by and the case was brought to my attention once again by Dr. Williams at a professional meeting we both attended. The insurer sent him my report and asked him to comment on my findings.

"I bet that made you uncomfortable," I offered. To which he replied that it had. Dr. Williams also admitted that he had gotten the necessary treatment wrong, and he thanked me for fixing things. He did not rebut my findings, and upon further reflection, reversed his recommendation that only a brief course of therapy was warranted. The end result was that a horrible event that changed someone's life resulted in a court order for adequate treatment. I had helped those involved in Janet's case feel a bit of her pain by using my colleague as a foil. I personally provided no treatment in this case, but I made sure that a reasonable amount of care would be guaranteed.

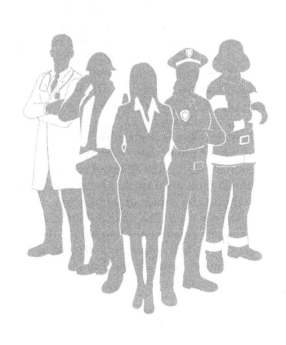

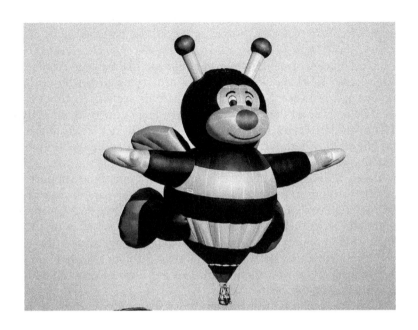

22 | On Being Chubby

There are far worse things than being short and overweight as a kid. I understand that I wasn't crippled, blind, or deaf. It was tough to be other than chubby, given my mom's Italian cooking. Homemade pizza, lasagna, Italian sausage, meatballs, and garlic bread. There was no "light cuisine" in our home. Rather, there was an abundance of food that symbolized prosperity and love. As they say in my mother's native language, "Mangia, mangia, mangia." Life was good.

Behavioral scientists tell us that primates discriminate based upon appearance within their species. Other mammals also pick mates by giving attention to "looks." It's been demonstrated that there are characteristics that birds look for among other birds, what snakes find attractive about other snakes, and even what unicellular organisms seek out in their own kind. It should not be a surprise that short, fat guys are at a distinct disadvantage for getting a date.

In the 1950s and 1960s, television helped shape our collective visions of what was America. Some supported the popular myth of the television show *Ozzie and Harriett*. In my family, *The Honeymooners* was considered more representative of what life was like for post-World War II Americans. Working-class stiffs were just trying to get by on hard work and perseverance. Sometimes, my parents argued. At times it got noisy. The cops never ended up at our door. Here's the deal, all of these ex-GIs assimilated back into normal life. Their brides let go of the responsibilities they had during the war. The country adapted, or at least we understood what was expected.

Being a short, fat kid was my fate. If my ma could support her family by working in a factory during her teenage years instead of excelling in high school, who was I to complain? If my dad got an all-expense-paid trip to Burma from Uncle Sam and some of his Army buddies didn't come back in one piece, what was my gripe? My point is, it's all relative. Compared to what folks go through elsewhere on this planet, during times of armed conflict or at points of economic hardship, what was my problem?

I didn't complain. I was shorter than my peer group, both the boys and girls, for years. I was said to be small, almost tiny. Yet my heft would argue against being truly tiny. One might describe me as pudgy in my preteen years. Being pudgy is not an endearing feature at that age. My paternal grandmother recognized my weight issue by noting that I had "boy boobs," a humiliating assessment which did not bring my father's mother and me closer together. That's just how Ethel was, straightforward and cruel. No wonder my dad left home at an early age.

Obesity is an epidemic in America. Obesity is officially defined as having a body-mass index (BMI) greater than 30. According to the Centers for Disease Control and Prevention (CDC) the prevalence (proportion or presence of a factor during a particular time period or at a certain point in time) of obesity among adult Americans was 42.4% in 2017-2018. Persons are considered overweight with a BMI of 25-29.9%; that designation applies to an additional 31% of adults. Thus, more than 70% of American adults have a weight problem. In 1999-2000, 30.5% of adults in our country were obese. In less than two decades, obesity in adults has gone from about 30% to over 42%. The trend is alarming. Having a weight problem begins early in life for many Americans. About 20% of adolescents and grade-school children are obese. Normal weight corresponds to a BMI less than 25, which is now the minority of adults in the United States.

Being overweight is associated with an increased risk for numerous health problems such as type 2 diabetes, hypertension, cardiovascular illness, osteoarthritis, and various types of cancer. Obesity is associated with decreased immune system functioning, lung capacity, and vaccine response. During the COVID-19 pandemic, obese Americans have been at greater risk for serious clinical presentations, hospitalization, and death. Genetics, environment, and social factors all contribute to why people become obese. For me as a kid, I loved to eat, my mom loved to cook, and my hormones had not kicked in yet. Bingo!

While acknowledging the chronic physical health problems associated with obesity, we must also recognize the adverse impact on one's psychological well-being. Self-image becomes problematic, and low self-esteem is common in folks with obesity. Pudgy kids are frequently bullied. Adults who are grossly obese are often discriminated against as job candidates or for promotion. It's embarrassing to ask for a larger chair or some type of accommodation due to body size. Years of being stared at, laughed at, and ridiculed due to one's appearance take a toll on the psyche.

Growing up, I can recall people who were overweight being referred to as "big boned." As a little kid, I thought it unusual that some people actually had more massive bone structure. It took me time to understand that this was just a euphemism for those who were plump or fat. I doubt anyone ever thought that being called "big boned" was a compliment. There are other euphemisms for being overweight. "She's a big girl. ...He's a stout fellow. ...That's quite the beer belly." These phrases call forth unattractive images and can cause emotional pain to those they are meant to describe.

There is an association between obesity and clinical depression. The obese have about a 25% increased risk for depression compared to those of normal weight. Persons who are depressed are also more likely to develop a weight problem. Teasing out cause and effect is challenging. For many, the weight issue develops insidiously along with features of depression, including sadness and low self-esteem. Recommendations for both conditions involve developing good habits regarding diet and vigorous exercise from an early age. Excessive television, cell phone and computer use; a diet of processed and fast food; and minimal amounts of regular physical exercise increase the chances for obesity and depression. Solutions exist for many so afflicted, but it takes conscious effort and commitment. I know that when I got away from the portions served at home and became involved in running, hiking, and bicycling, I lost weight and felt better physically and emotionally.

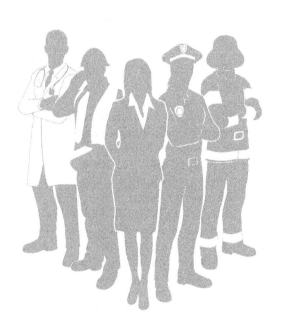

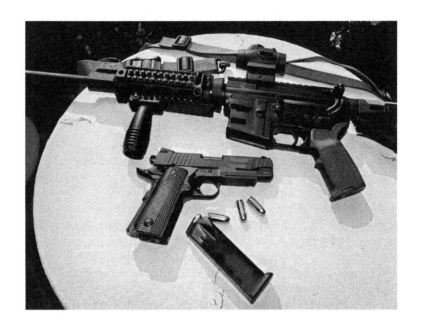

23 | We Have a Problem with Guns

Most people acknowledge there is a public health problem and/or epidemic of obesity in America. Gun violence is viewed differently, although it has also captured the attention of doctors and the general public. The statistics are impressive yet demoralizing. When using socioeconomic measures to assess quality of life across the globe, Americans do pretty well, with only a few other developed nations, such as Denmark and Japan, having slightly better rankings. Virtually all the countries with better socioeconomic statistics than the United States have nowhere near the gun violence problem seen in our country.

There are more guns owned by Americans than there are citizens. Each year, about 15,000 Americans are shot and killed by someone else, while another 23,000 use a firearm to commit suicide. Setting suicide aside, gunshot deaths result in a rate of more than 4 deaths per 100,000 population. That rate is nine times greater than for Canadians and 29 times higher than for the Japanese, according to the Gun Violence Archive. Americans are subjected to gun violence comparable to rates in unstable nations such as El Salvador where political unrest has been present for years and is similar to countries where gangs and drug cartels are battling with law enforcement. Socioeconomics alone does not explain why Americans are subjected to such high rates of death and injury from guns. What is clear is gun violence in America is a public health concern of epidemic proportion.

Nearly 40,000 Americans die from gunshot wounds each year. This includes homicide, suicide, self-defense, and accidents. Federal funding for research on gun violence has been restricted for two decades since a conservative Congress, backed by the National Rifle Association, intervened. After a study concluded that gun ownership increased the risk of a family member becoming a victim of gun violence, the gun lobby pushed for changes in federal law to prevent research funds from being used in a manner in which results could restrict gun rights. The weapons manufacturers won out, and our citizenry pays the price.

There are no accurate statistics on the number of people shot each year in the United States due to restrictions on federal funding of pertinent research. It is estimated that twice the number of victims who die approximates the number who are injured yet survive. Therefore, the total number of Americans shot each year is likely about 100,000. In a "good" month, there are 7,000 to 8,000 victims; in a "bad" month, the total is more than 10,000. That's more than 300 victims per day on average. A high price to pay for the right to bear arms.

Mass shootings, defined as resulting in the deaths of at least four victims, have become common in America. In 2018, our country experienced more mass shootings than the number of days in a year. Since the Las Vegas incident that took 58 lives in 2017, there have been mass shootings in Parkland, Florida; Pittsburgh, Pennsylvania; Thousand Oaks, California; and many more communities. Schools, places of worship, nightclubs, concerts, movie theaters, and other gatherings are potential slaughter sites. The answer to this phenomenon from gun rights advocates is more guns and increasing armed security. Is that really the kind of country we want?

Media dwells on mass shootings and gruesome accounts of killings using weapons. Survivors often have debilitating, life-altering injuries yet never come to the public's attention. Gunshot wounds to the head frequently result in brain injury and disfigurement. Victims with spinal cord injuries commonly live with nerve damage and paralysis for the remainder of their lives. The healthcare system responds by providing trauma surgery, intensive care, physical therapy, speech therapy, rehabilitation services, and mental health treatment, as though we were living in a war zone.

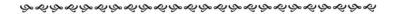

It was a lovely fall day in Chicago when I found myself the victim of an armed robbery. I had just met my future roommate. John and I crossed paths at the bulletin board posting housing options for medical students at Northwestern University. John had been living in a commune in Oregon and seemed overwhelmed by moving to a big city. He had also lost his dog and was having no luck recovering the pooch. While looking at prospective neighborhoods, we were approached by a young man who volunteered to educate us about communities on Chicago's Northside. After driving around for hours with our new acquaintance, we realized it was getting late. John offered to take the fellow to his home.

It was dark by the time we drove into the canyon of the Cabrini Green Housing Projects. Getting out of the car, I had a bad feeling about where we had ended up. Tall buildings surrounded us; landscaping was minimal to nonexistent. I noticed John was signing over traveler's checks. That didn't compute for me.

"John, what the heck are you doing?"

"Our friend said he wanted my money. When he pointed a gun at me, I told him all I had were the checks."

"Sign the checks, John," I responded.

While John stayed in the driver's seat signing over his savings, our robber friend got out and stood next to me. Before he could shake me down for what little cash I was carrying, a huge black dude walked by and gave him an ominous look.

"Shut up, man. That's a Stone," our robber told us emphatically. "Stone," as in Black P. Stone Nation, one of the more notorious gangs of Chicago. The robber had violated neighborhood rules by bringing two white guys into the 'hood. This was not allowed, even if the intent was to steal from them.

"Hey, man, take the gun. You shoot the brother." This inept criminal was now proposing that I take the handgun and get rid of the gang member! I recall jumping back into the passenger's seat and telling John to take off. I think we both expected to hear gunfire, which never came about. That was the last time either John or I visited Cabrini Green, which has since been destroyed. The incident gave me some insight into how screwed up situations can get when a gun is introduced.

Throughout my medical school and residency training, I was exposed to victims of gun violence. To this day and since developing a practice involving workplace issues, I commonly have had cases referred of working people involved in critical incidents where guns are used. Some have been bank tellers threatened at gunpoint. One was the convenience store clerk who was raped with a handgun for more than two hours. A number were paramedics who responded to trauma scenes involving shootouts. Of course, there have also been members of law enforcement who put on a vest to go to work and end up being shot at and returning fire.

∽❧∽❧∽❧∽❧∽❧∽❧∽❧∽❧∽❧∽❧∽❧

Aamir was a 42-year-old immigrant from Afghanistan. He came to live in California with his family at an early age. He did well in the public school system and went on to take college course work. After receiving an associate's degree in criminal justice, he applied to police departments in the Bay Area. He completed his police academy training after being accepted as a member of the Oakland Police Department. Throughout a career of more than a dozen years, Aamir was assigned primarily to patrol duties. Like his peer group, he worked different shifts throughout an urban landscape that included industrial areas, commercial zones, high-end residential neighborhoods, and ghettoes. He was physically fit and had a reputation with other cops as a standup kind of guy.

A woman had filed a complaint with the police, alleging that her boyfriend had brutally raped and beaten her. A medical exam and rape kit were conducted. A preliminary investigation concluded that there was probable cause to arrest the boyfriend. Aamir arrived down the street from where the suspect was known to reside. Another officer was in a separate vehicle at the other end of the block. A young adult male ran back into a residence next to the suspect's. Seconds later, the suspect emerged from his home armed with an AK-47 assault rifle. He got off a volley of fire, having been alerted to the officers' presence. Aamir, with gun drawn, took a round in his hip. The suspect proceeded to light up the squad cars.

While a call went out for backup from other police units in the area, Aamir crawled to the side of the building away from where the suspect had been shooting. It was dark, yet in the dim light, Aamir soon saw the suspect burst out of a side door, yelling, "Come kill me, you motherf***ers." He still had the AK-47. If he saw the officer, it would be all over for Aamir. The officer took aim while he lay bleeding on the pavement. Later he recalled thinking at the time, "Is this a justifiable shot?" Then he fired four times, hitting his target with three rounds that ended the alleged rapist's life.

Aamir and I met the next year. He had been taken to the local trauma center, where he underwent surgery for the gunshot that had fractured his hip, torn through tissue and blood vessels, and damaged nerves. While he still presented as a muscular man in his early 40s, there was a noticeable limp due to a permanent foot drop. He was also left with chronic pain in the low back, hip and leg. His career was over, and he knew vigorous activity such as running would never be possible. During many of his days and nights, while recovering from his physical injuries, he relived the shootout.

Aamir was grateful for the support of his department. He also had a loving family who was glad he had made it. He accepted that his life had changed irreparably. He had no guilt about the outcome. He didn't regret having pursued law enforcement as a career. He realized he could benefit from more counseling, but he felt he'd be better off not revisiting the incident. When we met, he was considering his options for alternative employment, as he was determined to be productive and a model for his children. More than ever, Aamir had a sense of pride as an immigrant who had been of service to his new homeland.

There are so many stories like Aamir's. Stories of careers being ended. Stories of lives lost. Stories of victims surviving only to live with scars and disabilities forever reminding them of the event that changed their lives. It is those stories that should cause persons of goodwill to speak out and stand up to the notion that our country's Second Amendment allows for the unfettered right to weaponry that is meant for the battlefield. Hopefully someday things will change. Enough is enough.

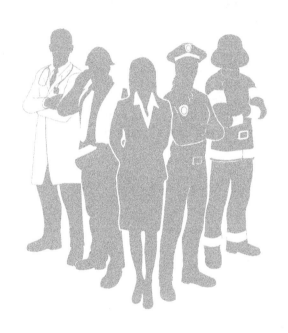

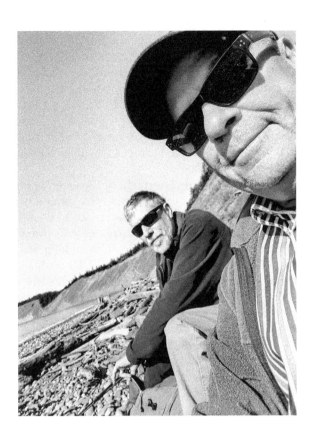

24 | Old Friends

Acareer involves time as a student, trainee, or apprentice, followed by work as employee, manager, or professional. In one's quest to attain a body of knowledge, a skill set, and a level of competence, it helps to have support from friends and family. As important as work is to establishing a person's identity, other elements of life matter as well. Friendship plays a role in maintaining a balanced existence. We often have little choice about members of our family. We may also have limited say over our co-workers. Friendships, though, develop over time while a mutual kinship is fostered. If we are lucky, some friends become old friends.

My best friend growing up was my brother Guy. He is two years younger, but was always a bit older than his chronologic age. Our close ties formed during family trips with our parents and when we were left at home to play together. In the summer months, we rode our bikes and played baseball. In the winter, we ice-skated and played hockey. We were given chores, which we shared, like mowing the lawn. We were embarrassed when our mother bought us clothes that gave the impression to others that we were twins. We both played in the school band. We shared some of the same friends, at least before our college years. We got our first paying jobs at the Farmer's Daughter Restaurant where Guy was hired first, when underage.

When I went off to college, I don't think I realized how I was abandoning my brother. He was left to live at home without a peer. It would be two years before Guy would go to college and be on his own. In the meantime, we wrote letters, since telephone calls were too expensive. During my freshman year in Boulder, Colorado, it was Guy who I turned to for help. I needed $50 to cover a fine for malicious mischief, a prank that was ill-advised. I couldn't ask my parents to assist without getting into more trouble, so I went to my best friend, who had my back. Of course, my parents found out, and I had to work seven days a week through the next summer, at two jobs, to restore their support for me returning to CU. Guy had come through.

As the years went by, the two of us took different paths. I pursued a career in medicine; Guy went into business. We both married and had kids. We lived in different parts of the country, but kept in touch. I appreciated his emotional support while I was going through tough times in my first marriage, which ended in divorce. Some years later, a rift developed in our relationship while his marriage was coming to an end. He let me know he didn't want my advice. Perhaps he again felt abandoned. Perhaps he felt talked down to. Perhaps he no longer needed advice from his older brother. Life is long, and my hope is that we can once again be friends.

I had other friends growing up. Some of us became members of our self-titled Black Marauders. We worked together at the Farmer's Daughter Restaurant and would go off, usually after work, and engage in antisocial acts such as driving on the local golf course after a snowstorm. Guy and I participated with fellow Marauders in putting For Sale signs in front of people's homes or filling a neighbor's lawn with reflective poles, which we termed "poomps." Somehow, we never got caught.

Tom, Bruce, and Mark were part of that group. At a 20-year high school reunion, Tom remarked on how dumb — and lucky — we had been as teens. At another reunion, 20 years later, Bruce refused to shake my hand. He apparently felt insulted by my political views. While I had protested the Vietnam War, Bruce later joined up and served our country as a member of the U.S. Army. I felt terrible about having somehow hurt this friend. I was unsure as to what I had said that caused the problem, so I consulted with Mark, who also was retired military.

Five years later at our 45-year reunion, Bruce and I had a sit-down chat and worked things out. Mark had spoken to Bruce, asking him to give me another chance. I learned a lot about Bruce on that occasion. I had not appreciated how tough his childhood had been. We made up and had expected to see each other at our 50-year reunion. I recently learned that Bruce died alone. That sad news reinforced for me the importance of making amends while one can.

Another Mark came along in med school. We were partners from our first day in anatomy lab. Three of the four of us assigned to the same cadaver would became psychiatrists. None of us had any intention of becoming shrinks when we applied to medical school. Mark and I became Californians. He ended up in the southern part of the state; I ended up in the north. Mark took on the role of godfather for my son, Henry. Mark, like my brother Guy, saw me through my divorce. We have stayed close friends for more than forty years. We both have had careers where legal issues are prominent. We share a view that along with tragedy, there can also come resilience. Maybe our senses of humor have helped sustain our friendship as well.

My friend Richard entered my life when I was in my late 30s. He's a cat with 12 lives. He traveled the world after leaving the Marines Corps. He worked in various jobs, some of dubious legality. For more than two decades, Richard has run a bar in California's Sonoma County. If you want to hear some stories, sit for an hour with Richard. Our bond was cemented at Giants games, Rolling Stones concerts, and playing pool at his bar. Richard commonly introduces me as his personal shrink, which others who know him find amusing, as he would never seek out mental health services. His barroom clientele is on the rough side — not all of them have all their teeth. Whenever I've been at Richard's bar and a band is playing, the place is jumpin'. What I most admire about Richard is his generosity and how he extends himself to others. He routinely sponsors fundraisers in his community for those in need.

Recently, a long-term friendship has been rekindled. Buzz and I met when we were 5. Our homes were within walking distance. We both remember pulling our pants down to show each other our penises. Boys! His family moved farther away, and while we both attended the same public schools, we ran in different circles. He played basketball while I was a Mathlete. Ironically, we were the only students in our graduating class from Carl Sandburg High School who enrolled at the University of Colorado. We were roommates for two and a half years before Buzz transferred to the University of Washington to study environmental design. We lost touch until recently. Buzz ended up in banking, which I never would have predicted. We had kids. We are both blessed with loving wives. Buzz and I share similar politics and a love of nature. His friendship dating back six decades does something simple and basic. It makes me happy. That's what friends are for.

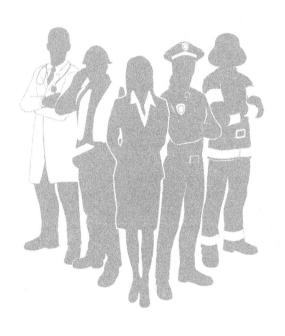

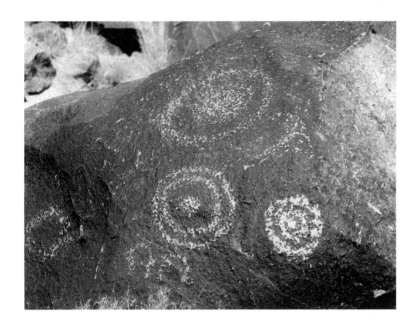

25 | Psychological Testing

Believe it or not, psychometric assessment began many centuries ago. More than four 4,000 years ago, the emperor of China used tests to periodically assess public officials. Ancient Babylonians, followed by the Greeks, used astrology to predict the future. Hippocrates and Plato developed understandings of illness and work. Then, during the Middle Ages, science and philosophy were neglected. By the mid-16th century, however, those fields of study were reborn during the Renaissance. In the late 18th century, the writings of Descartes introduced the concept of a mind-body dualism.

In 1895, American psychologist James McKeen Cattell proposed the idea of mental testing. Personality as a construct began with

Freud's *The Interpretation of Dreams*. The Binet-Simon Intelligence Scale was developed in France in the early 20th century. In 1921 the Swiss psychologist Hermann Rorschach wrote the book *Psychodiagnostik* that documented his studies. His book, published posthumously, was the basis for the projective psychological test known as the inkblot test, or the Rorschach. In 1939, the Weschler-Bellevue Intelligence scale was published, followed by the Weschler Adult Intelligence Test in 1955. Probably the most widely utilized measure of psychopathology, the Minnesota Multiphasic Personality Inventory (MMPI), was introduced in 1943. Since then, mental health practitioners have relied upon psychological tests to augment clinical opinions about the behavior, personality, and thinking of our fellow humans.

In my undergraduate training, I took three semesters of calculus as a component of my studies in science. To obtain a master's degree in public health, I was required to study statistics, which was beyond dry. During the four years of my psychiatric residency, I had not one didactic course on psychometrics. Psychologists were members of the faculty, but their role was primarily to supervise physicians-in-training on clinical cases. As a result, my peer group and I completed our psychiatric training with virtually no appreciation for the value and use of psychological testing.

In medical school, we learned to follow quantitative assessments such as complete blood counts, urinalysis, and pulmonary function studies because they were pertinent to the diagnosis and care of our patients. I don't recall ever having a supervisor during my psychiatric training suggest that psychological testing could be an important element of case formulation. I attribute this to a kind of ignorance or arrogance on the part of physicians, who at times undervalue what their non-medical colleagues have to offer.

The Briggs-Myers Type Indicator (MBTI) was published in 1962. This assessment of personal preferences has been widely used by employment consultants. The MBTI even helped select U.S. astronauts from candidate pools. Psychological testing is used in jurisdictions around the country to screen candidates for law enforcement. Typically, a battery of tests is administered to reduce the chances that an individual selected will later manifest problematic behavior, either during training or as an officer. One goal is to minimize the possibility of an officer becoming psychotic. No department wants an individual who is delusional or paranoid carrying a gun.

Candidates with anger issues, who have problems with authority, or who cannot make command decisions due to underlying anxiety should also be screened out. Currently, screening of police officer candidates in California selects those who are dependable, have good impulse control, are team players, are willing to take control of dangerous situations, wish to serve others, exert proper judgment, and tolerate stressful conflict, among other desirable attributes. Many other fields use some form of psychometric assessment when considering candidates for prospective employment. This is especially true when the cost of training, or the risk of failure once hired, is high.

During my first few years in practice, I experimented with traditional models by which psychiatrists provide their services. For five years, I worked part time at the county hospital in Oakland. I was good at emergency psychiatry or crisis intervention but came to see how one was likely to burn out taking care of persons in acute need. It's called the revolving door for a reason, and I did not have the temperament for a career dealing with a population of the severely mentally ill. Inpatient psychiatry had come to emphasize managing a patient's symptoms through medication. Not my cup of tea either. On the other end of the spectrum is the outpatient psychiatric practice, which I saw as a lonely path where the doctor spends his days providing individual counsel to patients, while having minimal contact with non-patients. For me conducting comprehensive consultation on cases with complex administrative, clinical, and legal components was a better fit with my scientific, medical, and public health background.

As I networked (before the term was used) in the San Francisco medical community, an opportunity arose. I was recruited to perform psychiatric evaluations at St. Francis Memorial Hospital of employees with stress claims. Four doctors from the medical specialties of internal medicine, orthopedics, physical medicine, and neurology ran the program. I learned a great deal in the years I worked with those colleagues. I had found my niche and came to slowly grow my own sources of referral outside of that program.

While grateful for the experience at St. Francis, it eventually was time for me to move on. In 1985, I took the risk of signing a three-year lease on office space in the financial district of San Francisco. I made a conscious choice to locate to a part of town where doctors were not usually seen. I also was disinterested in continuing to work in medical settings. If I were to focus on the issues of work and career, I wanted to be around working people.

Dr. Eric Morgenthaler was a young psychologist who came to my attention as I was about to start the medical group that came to be known as the Center for Occupational Psychiatry. Eric was also a Midwesterner, having grown up in Wisconsin. We met through evaluating work-related injury claims referred to a medical center in San Francisco. I was impressed with Eric's credentials but more so with his humanity. While dispassionate in his analysis of a person's psychological test results, he cared about how people were treated. Our budding connection led to my introduction to Dr. Harvey Lerchin, a psychiatrist who was interested in working with my new group. The three of us would work together for many years. After graduating from the University of Wisconsin, Eric received his doctorate from the California School of Professional Psychology in the Bay Area. He completed his post-doctoral training at a medical center in San Francisco and was ripe for the career option I offered him. It became a win-win situation. To this day, Dr. Morgenthaler and the Center continue to collaborate, while he and I remain friends.

Psychological testing is a major component of the psychiatric assessments conducted by our medical group. Many of my colleagues with clinical practices never request psychological tests of their patients. They instead rely upon their own diagnostic skills and whatever the patient's history provides. At the Center, we receive a substantial amount of information contained in medical and psychiatric records, as well as in personnel files, court documents, deposition transcripts, scholastic and military records, and sources not typically available to treating doctors. We don't have the luxury of conducting dozens of sessions with persons who come to our offices, so we need to obtain relevant data in ways that mental health practitioners usually do not access. Testing is a major component.

Over the years, Eric, with some input from me, developed a battery of standardized tests given to examinees at the Center. This included a screening measure of intelligence, a personality inventory, a questionnaire involving medical and psychiatric symptoms, a depression inventory, and a projective test, something like the Rorschach. Modifications are made to the testing, depending on the individual limitations of the person being evaluated. The tests require a person to have the academic skills of at least a sixth grader. The testing part of the evaluation typically takes from ninety minutes to three hours to complete, with breaks allowed. Eric produces a test report based upon the data that addresses questions from the evaluating psychiatrist. Those findings are then incorporated into the comprehensive psychiatric evaluation report issued to the referral sources in each case.

Sometimes more-complex testing is necessary, especially when there is concern that a brain injury has occurred. In those situations, Dr. Morgenthaler conducted neuropsychological testing that involved meeting directly with the examinee for most of a work day. Such testing allowed for increased accuracy regarding diagnosis, the nature and extent of cognitive impairment, and the prognosis for recovery. For many victims of mild head injury, brain scans might not demonstrate significant pathology though psychological testing can find areas of subtle, yet real abnormality. The following is a composite sketch of the type of case which required neuropsychological testing.

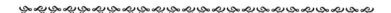

Mr. James was a 50-year-old divorced former professional football player referred by his attorney for evaluation related to claims of physical and mental injury. This retired athlete had experienced cumulative trauma associated with a 13-year career in the NFL for three teams. His claims included orthopedic injuries resulting in multiple surgeries to the knees, upper extremities, and low back. Those claims were evaluated by orthopedic experts.

Dr. Morgenthaler met with Mr. James and obtained additional relevant history. After completing his college education at a major university where he maintained a "B" average, he began his professional career with the Oakland Raiders, where for five seasons he was an offensive lineman. He later played for teams in Kansas City and Denver. In his years as a professional athlete, he had three documented concussions and many more instances where he was dazed and confused after physical contact during games and practice. He complained of memory problems, irritability, sleep difficulty, chronic headaches, outbursts of aggression, and a series of bad business decisions since retiring from football.

In addition to reviewing medical records, which included brain scans and neurologic consults, Dr. Morgenthaler conducted a clinical interview and administered a battery of psychological tests to address cognitive and psychological issues. These tests included the Wechsler Adult Intelligence Scale-IV, the Wechsler Memory Scale-IV, the California Verbal Learning Test-II, the Test of Premorbid Functioning, the ACS Effort Assessment, the Dot Counting Test, the Trail Making Test, the Letter Fluency Test, the Stroop Color and Word Test, the MMPI-2, and the Beck Depression and Anxiety Inventories.

Most notably, the test results demonstrated an individual of average intelligence who was experiencing mild impairment in visual and verbal memory, moderate impairment in complex drawing reproduction and visuomotor integration, moderate impairment in organization and planning, mild to moderate depression with a tendency toward outbursts of aggression, and mild anxiety with associated physical health concerns. His prognosis was guarded because there was a good chance his symptoms would progress with time.

A cognitive disorder was diagnosed and attributed to cumulative industrial injury from episodes of closed head trauma. Recommendations included a repeat brain scan and neurologic consultation to address post-concussive headaches. Mr. James was expected to have persistent problems with memory, judgment, and problem solving, as well as with activities of daily living.

The value of psychological testing rests in providing a quantitative assessment of cognitive and psychological functioning, allowing for comparison of an individual's performance over time. Standard test measures with established validity are used. Rather than rely solely upon the client's subjective complaints, the clinician can consider additional quantitative scores and norms when addressing the issues of diagnosis, disability, treatment, and rehabilitation in persons presenting with psychiatric conditions. As in the case of Mr. James, test performance over time can lead to modification of treatment and supportive measures. Perhaps in the future, biological measures of psychological functioning that go beyond currently available brain scans will augment what science now provides.

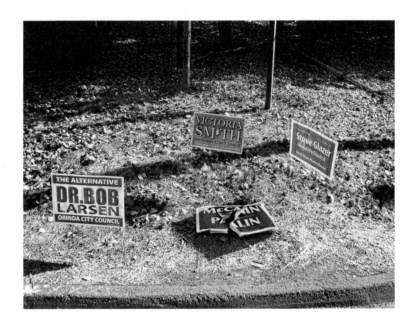

26 | It Comes Down to Politics

Growing up, I knew my parents were registered Republicans. They were the kind of voters who were fiscally responsible, supported public education, wanted an effective military, expected the roads to be paved, and were disinterested in their neighbors' personal lives. Today they'd probably be Democrats.

While some of my high school peers were interested in running for student council, that didn't appeal to me. By the time I got to college in Boulder, Colorado, I was focused on bigger things. It was impossible for me not to pay attention to the positions political leaders in America were taking on the Vietnam War, women's issues, civil rights, and a plethora of topics that brought many together while alienating younger voters from the establishment.

My father and I had numerous, contentious discussions about the state of our nation during the 1970s. Like many young adults at the time, I viewed the Nixon administration with mistrust. Like college students across the country, undergraduates in Boulder marched against the war. We also protested nuclear arms and radioactive waste. While working in support of the McGovern campaign in 1972, I felt justified in voting down the Winter Olympics out of environmental concerns and in voting for the Equal Rights Amendment (ERA). The arguments against the ERA were that America would end up with unisex bathrooms and female combatants in the military. Ironically, our nation has yet to ratify the ERA, but the predicted social changes have nevertheless occurred.

Dad called me a "bad loser" when Nixon was reelected. "I AM a bad loser, but I am not just a bad loser. He cheated." I was told to get over it. As the Watergate hearings concluded and members of Nixon's staff headed off to federal prison terms, my father grudgingly admitted that a fair amount of cheating and bad behavior had taken place. Life went on, Nixon resigned, and the war eventually ended in 1975. It was a tumultuous time for the country.

My interest in politics died down during medical school. After all, there were nerve pathways to memorize and physiologic processes to grapple with. My priorities had changed, and I needed a rest from the conflict the war years had fostered abroad and at home. What would I do with all the information about bodily mechanisms I was assimilating? Would I become a family doctor? Was there still a place for me as a research physician? Did I have the skills to be a surgeon? Where might this developing interest in mental disorders and human behavior lead me?

During 1978, my internship year in San Francisco, several major events took place that captured the public's attention. The mass suicide at Jonestown in Guyana had close ties to the Bay Area through the cult's leader, Jim Jones. Then Mayor George Moscone and Supervisor Harvey Milk were assassinated by disgruntled Supervisor Dan White. It was a dark time in San Francisco. The White Night Riots followed White's acquittal, as the media portrayed him as getting away with murder with his using the "Twinkie defense." My family was convinced that I had moved to the modern day version of Sodom and Gomorrah.

Diane Feinstein became the mayor of San Francisco as a result of Moscone's death. As a physician-in-training and representative of the San Francisco Medical Society, I met privately with Mayor Feinstein to discuss public health issues. Her first husband had been a physician, and I recall Mayor Feinstein being very cordial to me as an early-career doctor. Years later, during her initial campaign for the U.S. Senate, I supported her with a campaign contribution, which was in turn recognized by my receiving a distinctive lapel pin. So that's how this political stuff works!

My renewed interest in politics came about through a desire to support public policy measures dealing with health care. Along with involvement in local and state medical associations, I was elected by the membership as a resident councilor of the Northern California Psychiatric Association (NCPS). Through the NCPS, I spoke out in support of the ERA when the national psychiatric organization changed policy and decided to have its annual meeting in New Orleans, despite Louisiana not having passed the ERA. (Previously, the American Psychiatric Association's policy was to hold meetings only in states that had ratified the ERA.)

As a trainee, I became involved with professional associations and the state licensing board in identifying and assisting "impaired" physicians. The argument for rehabilitation of professionals goes like this: Punishment might get rid of the bad apples, but the cost is high to the individual physician and potentially to patients who could have benefitted from services provided if the licensee had been rehabilitated. Physicians, attorneys, dentists, police officers, firefighters, and others providing service to the public might be seen as a community resource. Our society hopes to recoup its investment in these professionals over the course of a long career. If the premature ending of a professional's career is averted, it has the potential to benefit the provider of services and the public.

My experience with impaired doctors made it clear to me that these cases are not subtle. Often, the central issue involves alcohol or substance abuse. Not uncommonly, access to controlled substances is too attractive for some doctors to resist. Anesthesiologists, as a group, have a high rate of prescription drug use, in part because they have easy access to opioids and other highly addictive drugs. State licensing boards work in conjunction with professional associations to give the addicted and/or mentally disturbed licensee an alternative to disciplinary action. If mutually agreeable, the doctor or attorney is "diverted" into a program of treatment that monitors one's progress and allows for continued practice within specified guidelines. By my assessment, this is a win-win situation.

What does it take for a professional to become recognized as impaired? A licensing board, such as the State Bar of California or the Medical Board of California, becomes involved in an attorney's or a doctor's case when the bar or board are concerned the public is at risk. After all, most of us don't want a drunken attorney or an intravenous drug-abusing physician providing services to our family. Addicted doctors, pharmacists, and nurses can steal medication for personal use. Attorneys and accountants are more likely to commit fraud when they need money to help supply their drug of choice.

Aside from substance abuse, impairment can involve gambling losses, reckless business decisions, or a pattern of marital and relationship disasters. The scenarios are not pretty. However, if caught in time and they are amenable to change their behavior, such professionals can be helped as they have much to lose. Working with impaired doctors required me to be an advocate for folks who at times were highly unlikable. When you believe in public policy to save these souls, then intervention is necessary to stave off license revocation while the individual is given a second chance.

Fortune intervened when I first became involved with the California Society for Industrial Medicine and Surgery (CSIMS). I was almost 40 when I was elected by my peers as their president. CSIMS is a statewide occupational medicine association involved in lobbying for medical practice issues while also advocating for patients' rights. Members provide evaluation and treatment to workers injured on the job, including those with mental as well as physical injuries. Needless to say, the employer and insurer communities do not always see things the same way as do employees and their doctors. Not uncommonly, I found myself testifying before legislative committees in Sacramento or meeting with assembly members and state senators to educate them about conditions they might not well appreciate. Unfortunately, cost concerns have resulted in limits placed on the type of injuries found to be compensable. Yet good public policy on industrial injuries considers not only economics, but also science and beliefs about what workers deserve.

If a convenience store clerk is raped while covering the night shift, no one would question whether that employee had been physically injured. Would we also see her as having incurred a mental injury, which could result in the need for treatment? Violent acts might or might not result in physical injury. Does a bank teller subjected to multiple robberies not deserve recognition of her post-traumatic stress in the form of counseling and perhaps an alternative job assignment? Should a police officer who shoots and kills an armed felon committing a violent crime not have access to a psychologist, if desired? Workers' compensation systems vary enormously across states as to how such claims are handled. My advocacy over almost three decades has been to stand up for workers with legitimate mental problems brought forth by just doing their jobs.

This interest in advocacy for employees with both physical and mental conditions related to employment led to my being a member of the Industrial Medical Council (IMC) in California for 13 years. I was appointed by Sen. David Roberti, president pro tem of the state Senate. As the psychiatric representative to the IMC, I worked with my colleagues in orthopedics, internal medicine, physical medicine, neurology, chiropractic, psychology, and other relevant clinical specialties to establish guidelines for the evaluation and treatment of claimants with industrial injuries. Trust me when I say that politics was omnipresent in that process. This is a multibillion-dollar business in California. It is expensive to adjudicate injury claims and provide appropriate benefits.

In the fields of psychiatry and psychology, we held hearings that resulted in curtailing abusive practices in the evaluation of mental injury claims. Doctors could no longer use clerical staff to interview patients or summarize records. Many clinicians were upset about that change. Too bad. A simple schedule was established for psychological testing, eliminating excessive and unnecessary practices. Again, certain colleagues were displeased. Treatment guidelines were established to address what should be provided to employees suffering from PTSD. Consultants from major universities including UCSF, UCLA, and Duke University, contributed to the science considered by the committee of clinicians that developed the final guidelines.

My own venture as a candidate for political office came when I reluctantly entered the race for City Council in a Bay Area community. I was up against fellow Democrats who were incumbents — a political consultant and a real estate attorney. My campaign slogan was "Dr. Bob: The Alternative." When I challenged the other candidates to take no contributions from entities doing business with our city, they turned me down. I, of course, supported the city employees' demand to receive pension benefits. I also wanted to maintain and support our police force.

My problem was that I publicly criticized the school board's oversight of bond funds intended to fix the infrastructure of local high schools, which never happened. Despite being a professor at a state university, I was labeled as an evil person who opposed the funding of public schools! My wife was thrilled that I lost the election, given the prospect of me fighting against real estate developers for the next four years. I take perverse pride in viewing myself as a "supporter of losing-but-just causes." In this last particular case, it was my own campaign.

I remain involved in politics to this day. I frequently write letters to the editor of our local newspaper on access to care, mental health topics, and public health and safety concerns. I also testify before state legislative committees on gun safety issues. The COVID-19 pandemic has demonstrated the complex interactions between politics, science, and public policy in our nation and across the globe where achieving consensus is often difficult. In the end, it comes down to politics, like it or not.

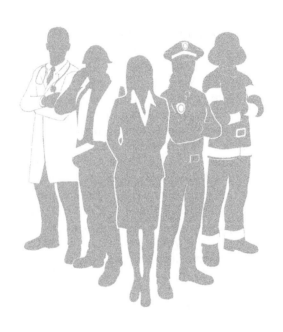

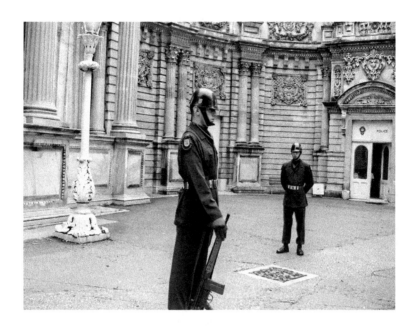

27 | Fit for Duty

State and federal laws allow for clinical evaluation of employees under certain circumstances. Prospective employees being considered for a job position might be asked to submit to drug screening. Jobs where safety issues arise might permit random drug screening of workers. For example, commercial drivers and transit operators often are expected to submit urine samples for evidence of illicit or prescription drugs that could affect the operation of a motor vehicle. A medical examination might also be required before an individual is hired to assure the employer that the prospect can handle the demands of the job.

Professional athletes typically undergo a physical examination by a team-appointed physician before an agreed-upon contract is finalized.

Candidates for jobs in law enforcement undergo psychological testing and a clinical interview, in addition to background checks. Departments want to avoid hiring and training an officer who has problems with authority, is excessively angry, has unusual beliefs, or cannot make command decisions. These assessments of physical and mental function are termed "fitness for duty" examinations.

No one likes psychiatric fitness-for-duty evaluations. The employee sees the process as intrusive. The employer would rather not have concerns about an individual's state of mind. The clinician must be careful to maintain neutrality so as not to be viewed as either an advocate of the interviewee or the employer. Unlike the doctor-patient relationship that most of us are familiar with, there is no confidentiality when the individual being referred for assessment agrees to proceed with the requested examination. In this chapter, we consider the behavior, actions, and performance that might cause an employee to be evaluated for psychological fitness to perform the duties of a particular job. All of the cases portrayed are of workers who were causing disruption in the workplace or toward the public. In each case, a determination had to be made if the worker could continue to be employed and under what circumstances.

༄ ༄ ༄ ༄ ༄ ༄ ༄ ༄ ༄ ༄ ༄ ༄ ༄ ༄

Ms. Greene was a middle-aged employee of a municipality north of San Francisco whose job was to counsel youths in inner city neighborhoods. She had demonstrated erratic behavior and moodiness on multiple occasions in the past six months. By then, she had been working in her outreach position in the community for several years. On one occasion, she stopped her city vehicle, exited the car, and jumped between two groups of young adults who were brandishing firearms. Rather than call the police, she chose to intervene on her own by shouting at the two groups. Local police arrived shortly after the confrontation had begun and essentially were required to rescue Ms. Greene from the highly volatile situation.

Arrests were made and the outreach worker was questioned by the responding officers. Ms. Greene received a written disciplinary action from the employer in the form of a warning for having violated procedure. She in turn filed a grievance through her union for harassment on the part of the police and her manager. She was convinced she had acted properly. In an unusual development, a statement from one of the persons arrested for illegal possession of a firearm referred to her as "that crazy bitch who almost got herself killed."

The following month, Ms. Greene threatened to jump from a moving vehicle. She was riding with a co-worker to make a home visit at a youth center when an argument ensued over their working relationship. While the vehicle was moving quickly on a freeway, Ms. Greene took off her seat belt and cracked open the passenger-side door. Though she responded to the driver's plea to shut the door, she continued to berate her co-worker until they arrived at their destination. Even so, she exited the car as it was still being parked. Refusing to apologize, she then left the area and returned on her own to the city offices, where she filed a complaint about her co-worker's alleged bad driving. An investigation took place, with Ms. Greene admitting to having opened the door of a moving vehicle. She also acknowledged that she had in the past leapt from a friend's car when she felt unsafe. She was given a two-day suspension for her actions. Her response was to again file a grievance through her union for harassment.

During the evaluation in our offices, Ms. Greene described herself as having a "strong personality." Having grown up in a tough neighborhood, she identified with many of the gang members in the community where she worked. She termed them "my homies," while speaking with disdain about co-workers she considered to be "ignorant about the streets." During her tenure with the city, she had filed a stress claim, though she never showed up for the scheduled psychological evaluation. Her work history included previous employment in a medical office and as an advocate in a youth program. Her parents, who were now deceased, had taken her to counseling during her "rebellious" teenage years.

After dropping out of high school, Ms. Greene lived in various locations while "doing every drug I could get my hands on." She received training that led to her job in a medical office. Married and divorced three times, she was currently living with a female partner. The only psychiatric care she had received as an adult was provided through her employer's employee assistance program (EAP). Psychometric testing was consistent with an individual with poor academic skills. More notably, she came across as manic, highly mistrustful, and delusional.

Ms. Greene was found unfit psychologically for her counseling position. Her erratic behavior with the public and co-workers was likely the expression of a bipolar disorder or some other psychotic illness. Left untreated, she would remain a safety concern for herself and others. The recommendation was for her to be placed on a six-month disability leave, during which she was expected to participate in outpatient psychiatric care that included individual and group psychotherapy, drug screening, and a trial of a mood stabilizer. Monthly treatment reports would be required, and when her treating clinicians determined she could return to work for the city, a reevaluation of her fitness should take place before her job was reinstated. Time would determine whether Ms. Greene might stabilize psychologically and resume her counseling duties.

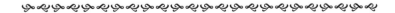

The case of Mr. Thomas involved a referral from a public school district where he had worked for three years as a high school science teacher. An experienced educator in his late 30s, he had moved to the community after marrying his current wife. He denied there were any particular problems in the marriage. He claimed it was "the imbeciles I work with" who sent him to our offices. From early on in his work at the high school, Mr. Thomas found himself disappointed with both the caliber of students and the faculty. His complaints were numerous.

Mr. Thomas described the chemistry lab as a mess when he started his first year. The biology teacher used up too much shared supplies. Mr. Thomas had to cover for the physics teacher on a regular basis. The administration wouldn't back him up when he gave failing grades to some of the "boneheads" he had to teach. Then, there were the parents who did nothing but complain that their kids had too much homework.

Mr. Thomas admitted that his "ranting" at the students had not worked. He contrasted his experience teaching with his having attended Catholic schools, where disrespect was not tolerated. By his second year, he felt shunned by his fellow teachers, which he attributed to their differing views regarding expectations for student performance. He continued to find himself in disagreements with other teachers. He insisted that he never threatened anyone, though he admitted that his presence at times might be imposing. Most recently, a number of complaints had come to the attention of the school administration about Mr. Thomas openly criticizing fellow teachers in front of students. After the principal met with him privately, Mr. Thomas agreed to see a local psychologist. He found those sessions helpful in dealing with his frustration.

Information from the school district described a teacher who was highly proficient, though prone to dramatic displays of emotion during discussions with faculty and administrators. His profuse sweating, facial contortions, and body movements concerned co-workers, who found him to be unduly critical and short-tempered. Psychometric test results were consistent with an individual of high intelligence who reported minimal emotional distress. However, his attention to detail was also associated with rigid standards and a tendency toward volatility in interactions with others. My evaluation concluded that Mr. Thomas had no serious mental illness. While technically capable of teaching high school, it was probably a bad fit for him. The referral to the psychologist had allowed the teacher to consider alternative positions more in keeping with his character. My evaluation found Mr. Thomas fit to complete the school year. He planned to finish up at the high school and then return to teach at a community college, where the pay was less but where he hoped he would not feel undermined. If for some reason he returned to the high school, additional sessions with his psychologist would be advisable.

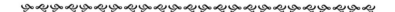

Ms. Choi had worked for almost 10 years at a five-star hotel in San Francisco when she came to our offices. She was in her late 40s and had worked in a number of food service positions. Human resources had received complaints from co-workers about Ms. Choi voicing unusual thoughts to them on a number of occasions. Management did not know what to make of it when she reported during a meeting that "creatures" roamed the hallways of the hotel late at night. Ms. Choi was glad to see that the company was finally taking her seriously after she had gone to building security about these incidents.

The creatures allegedly resembled a female guest who was kept in a basement freezer at the hotel. Ms. Choi wondered why other employees seemed unaware of a ghost in room 1205, who she had heard speak in some strange European language. Ever since she had been trapped in a service elevator with a dead body while working room service eight years ago, more and more creepy things had happened. (There was no indication the employee had actually been trapped anywhere with a dead body.) No one seemed to be bothered, so she mostly kept these episodes to herself.

Ms. Choi's history included growing up in an intact working-class family in a capital city in Asia. She completed the equivalent of high school and took additional training that led to her working in cafeterias and as a cashier. She denied having any particular traumas during her upbringing except for a grandmother who was quite harsh. At the age of 30, she came with family to live in California. Her English skills were proficient enough that she took a job working for a small hotel until she accepted her current employment, which came with union benefits. She had no chronic illnesses and prided herself on seldom taking a sick day. A few years prior, Ms. Choi had mentioned the ghost to her doctor. That physician prescribed medicine that made it difficult for her to get out of bed. That same physician later referred her to a counselor, but all that therapist wanted to do was talk about how the ghost and the creatures made Ms. Choi feel. "It was scary. So, I quit going. Things were OK for a while, but then I passed by the freezer with the dead lady again."

Ms. Choi presented her concerns about the scary visions in a matter-of-fact manner. Upon further questioning, she admitted that she had been visited by ghosts a long time ago, when she and her husband had been separated. The herbs she bought seemed to help back then. Psychological test results found her to experience hallucinations, paranoia, delusions, depression, and discomfort in interpersonal relations. My report confirmed the employer's concerns. Left untreated, Ms. Choi was unfit for work in food services, or any other service position in the hotel. While she did not represent a danger to herself or others, she would continue to make co-workers, and potentially guests, feel uncomfortable. Some of her beliefs had led to her discarding food that she mistakenly concluded had been poisoned by the hall creatures.

A referral for psychiatric treatment was recommended. A trial of an antipsychotic drug was in order. A medical workup should take place to eliminate the slim possibility that this worker's thoughts were the product of metabolic illness or a brain mass. With effective treatment that was predicted to be long-term, she could potentially resume her job at the hotel. If not, she should qualify for disability benefits. The long-term outcome in Ms. Choi's case was never reported to me, though our office was informed that co-workers felt relief when she was continued on a leave.

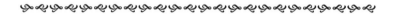

As is seen in these fitness-for-duty cases, it takes serious dysfunction to trigger such consultations. Mental illness can be disabling and painful. Mood swings, irrational beliefs, and recurrent conflict impact not only the individual workers, but also their co-workers, supervisors, and clients. While treatment is not always the answer, it most definitely has its place where avoidance and denial have failed. Recognizing psychopathology in a troubled employee is just as important as assisting a worker with a physical disability that otherwise interferes with productivity.

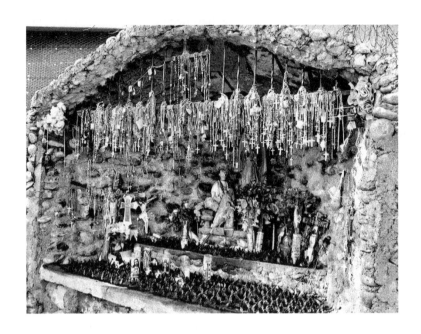

28 | Grieving the Loss

Many injured workers end up mourning what they have lost, sometimes multiple losses. My mother would say, "We don't appreciate our health until we don't have it anymore." How true. In my experience, we take our health for granted until we have a serious accident or illness. In medical school, I studied diseases with an esoteric interest, because heart disease and cancer seemed like distant risks. Having been a real patient in more recent times, I now have more appreciation for good health. I also understand what it's like to be scared about whether a course of treatment will work or not.

Ms. West was in her mid-50s. For two decades, she had been employed by the same school district from which she had graduated from high school. She was a teacher's aide, working with a special-needs population of students. Previously, she had been a nanny. She had children of her own and left the workforce when they were young. Following a divorce, she went to work in the public school system, as the idea of helping students learn and mature appealed to her. Initially, she was assigned duties in a grammar school setting, where she assisted special education teachers with young kids who had developmental disabilities, behavioral problems, and recognized mental disorders. She found the work challenging, though gratifying.

Over the years, Ms. West was exposed to kids throwing temper tantrums and worse. She had little formal training to differentiate a child with a recognized mental disorder, such as attention deficit disorder, from one who was merely neglected by their parents. She knew that timeouts had worked with her children when they did not obey, and that became part of her armamentarium in dealing with students who misbehaved. Her students were different from her daughters though, because these kids could become very angry and impulsive. She learned when it was best to separate students before they started hitting each other. At times, she got helpful suggestions from the teachers and a school psychologist.

The kids who ended up being mainstreamed into regular classes were the success stories. Some just grew up. Others benefited from medication, which allowed them to pay attention and not be disruptive. Some students' bad behavior escalated with time. Ms. West ended up on a leave of absence after a fourth grader threatened her with a knife that he had in his backpack, along with books and pencils. She hadn't been physically injured, but found herself nervous when returning to work. A physician prescribed medication to help her sleep. She transferred to another grade school, and her fears seemed to improve.

Ms. West then had an opportunity to work at the local high school. She knew a number of the teachers and administrators there, and she looked forward to being of service to an older group of students whom she could monitor and counsel. While some of the special-needs adolescents were like teddy bears, a more challenging subset could be volatile and provocative. Some of these teenagers were big and strong. Some had to be disciplined for being verbally abusive. She caught one older boy sneaking up behind her in an effort to look down her blouse. When she reported the incident, she was told, "Boys will be boys."

Facing no consequences for his actions, that teenager later exposed himself to her. The matter was documented, and the teen was suspended. He eventually returned to the same class, though another aide was assigned to work with him. Months went by before Ms. West suddenly realized she was alone with the boy during a break after other

144

students and staff had left the classroom. She described "freaking out" and directing him to leave. When she followed him into the hallway, he proceeded to masturbate in her presence. This episode resulted in the student again being suspended and, on this occasion, transferred to another campus.

Ms. West continued working at the high school, where she found herself routinely fearful. After another teenager threatened her life, she walked off the job and scheduled an appointment with her regular physician. The physician referred her to a psychologist, who placed his new patient on a disability leave. The physician also prescribed an antidepressant, a drug she did not like. Months into treatment, her psychologist described her as "precluded from returning to any assignment with students who had histories of serious behavioral problems." Her long-term employer responded by indicating there was no alternative assignment available. Ms. West's career was effectively over.

Her outpatient counseling ended. Her disability payments were reduced when her condition was no longer considered temporary. Once the school district found her ineligible for reemployment, her employment benefits, including health insurance, ended. Despite her lengthy service with the district, she was too young to receive anything more than partial retirement benefits. While relieved to know she didn't have to return to a setting she saw as unsafe, she missed the social contacts she had with co-workers. She found herself anxious when out in public, especially in the presence of strangers. She was at a loss when considering what type of work she might pursue. Going back to school at her age seemed daunting. While her male partner and adult daughters were supportive and understanding, Ms. West saw herself as weak and worthless. She described struggling with the emotions typical of a person who has lost a loved one.

What we see in the case of Ms. West is a worker who, as a result of bad experiences at work, became anxious, fearful, and mistrustful. While time away from the work setting and outpatient treatment helped her accept the recommendation to avoid interactions with disturbed teens, she considered herself to have been cast aside. She lost her job and had to figure out how to get by on reduced income and with no health insurance. Ms. West's friends were employed, which left her feeling lonely and useless. This was not the life she had envisioned for herself. She ended up fearful, dejected, and feeling powerless with regard to her future. It is as though she was consumed by grief.

❧❧❧❧❧❧❧❧❧❧❧❧❧❧❧❧❧

Not that many years ago, the California Legislature significantly reduced benefits to workers who experienced secondary psychiatric symptoms in response to having been physically injured. I found myself seated next to a 40-year-old member of the pipefitters' union during one of the hearings on this issue. I was in Sacramento awaiting my time to testify before an insurance committee of the California Assembly. The proposal was to eliminate permanent disability benefits for mental conditions resulting from industrial physical injuries. In the future, only employees with "catastrophic" injuries such as burn injuries, amputations, brain damage, and paralysis would be eligible for receiving additional disability benefits beyond what the physical disabilities might justify. My intention was to convince legislators that reducing benefits would not make such problems go away.

The pipefitter sitting beside me had been a skilled worker employed at a state university by a construction contractor. He was literally working in a hole in the ground to secure footings for a new building when a co-worker turned on machinery without notice. The pipefitter's non-dominant left hand was mangled despite his having worn gloves. He was taken by ambulance to a trauma center, where he underwent surgery to stop the bleeding and stabilize the damage to bones, nerves, muscles, and connective tissue. After two years and seven reconstructive hand surgeries, his left hand was essentially useless for tasks requiring gripping, grasping, and fine dexterity. He was taking pain medication and an anticonvulsant for his chronic nerve pain. No further surgery was recommended. He could not return to his profession.

Given his young age, it had been recommended that this pipefitter apply for Social Security disability benefits. In addition to his physical symptoms and limitations, he described suffering from insomnia, social withdrawal, sensitivity about the appearance of his damaged hand, irritability, and a sense of futility. He tried to contain his sobbing as he testified before the legislators, who listened respectfully. Everyone present was moved by the pipefitter's account. When he finished, I stated that no one should doubt that this man's life had been irreparably harmed by doing his job. It was also clear that he was suffering emotionally, in addition to his recognized physical injuries.

Unfortunately, the California Legislature voted nonetheless to limit benefits for psychiatric injuries that arise as a result of admitted physical injuries. Despite the power of the pipefitter's tale, the insurance industry, representing employers' interests, won out. Cost containment prevailed over establishing equity for employees struggling with psychological issues in addition to their physical problems. Legislators voting with the majority probably saw themselves as doing their jobs by being fiscally responsible. Perhaps they convinced themselves that workers like the pipefitter would still qualify for some benefits, as his injuries would be considered "catastrophic."

In reality, workers affected by this law have difficulty being recognized with injuries severe enough to justify acceptance of a psychiatric claim for additional benefits. The argument that usually prevails is that while a back injury requiring multiple surgeries or a crush injury that leaves the individual disfigured is terrible, such persons have not experienced a truly catastrophic event.

Like the medical student who takes his health for granted, the insurance industry lobbyists and many of our legislators have little understanding about how tenuous life can be. (A California Workers' Compensation Appeals Board decision published in 2019 addressed the concept of catastrophic injury. See Chapter Eight entitled "Burn, Baby, Burn," where psychological reactions to burn injuries were discussed.) Perhaps a more just society would recognize the complexity of the loss so many who are legitimately injured experience.

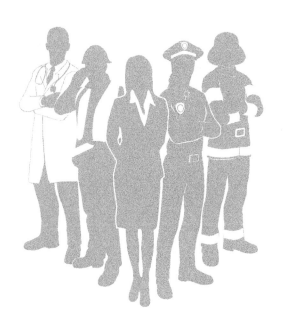

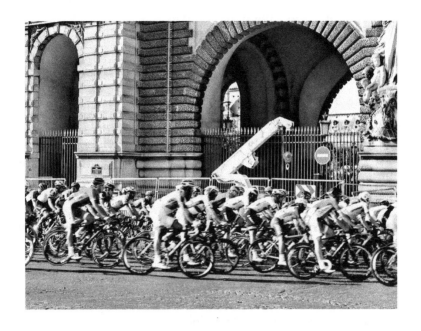

29 | We Don't Work Alone

There is no such thing as a self-made man. When it comes to goods produced and services delivered, it takes a village, or at least a team, to get the job done. My first real job as a busboy at the Farmer's Daughter Restaurant had me working with dishwashers, the janitor, the chef, his kitchen staff, waitresses, the hostess, and the maître d'. Two years later, as a teamster on a loading dock, I worked with other laborers, forklift drivers, truckers, machinists, production workers, supervisors and, of course, janitors. My college work-study job in Dr. Goldstein's laboratory exposed me to taking direction from professors who were scientists and from their postdoctoral fellows. If I worked late enough, I also had contact with janitors. It turns out that janitors are society's first line of defense against the second law of thermodynamics, which states that the world moves toward entropy or chaos on its own.

My first job in a hospital or medical center was working at Jackson Memorial Hospital in Miami for Dr. Wise, a cell biologist referenced in prior chapters. We worked in research laboratories affiliated with the University of Miami, School of Medicine. As this was the county hospital for Dade County and our lab was within the Department of Anatomy, the morgue was nearby. I found myself interacting with scientists, pathologists, orderlies, technicians, and a variety of clinical staff. There most definitely is a need for janitors and custodians in a place with sick patients and dead bodies. I went on to work as a research technician at university medical centers in Boston and Chicago. Janitors cleaned things up there as well. In my view, those men and women are the unsung heroes who allow the rest of us to get our work done. Many work the night shift long after most employees, except for the security guards, have gone home. By morning, the trash is gone, the toilets are clean, and the floors have been polished — a modern miracle that many of us take for granted. Perhaps as a result of the COVID-19 pandemic, these services are better appreciated.

After completing my psychiatric residency, I was fortunate to find office space in an old Victorian on California Street in San Francisco. Dr. Anderson, a psychiatrist, colleague, and good friend, was a partner in the building's ownership and has done quite well by investing in real estate. Frankly, though, working in an old, lovely structure designed to be a single-family residence had its limitations for conducting my business. My office was on the second floor, accessed by a long stairway. It was impossible to care for patients with significant physical disabilities in that lovely, yet antiquated, setting. The building had a waiting room, a bathroom, and a kitchen that also served as the central mail and message location. There was no room for office equipment. All of the building's occupants were male shrinks. Most were psychoanalysts and fatherly figures. None had a practice like the one I was developing. As my practice grew, it became apparent that I would need a more suitable office space. Eventually, the time came for me to move to a real office building.

When the Center for Occupational Psychiatry opened in 1985 in downtown San Francisco, it was a big move in many ways. The office building at 690 Market Street had survived the 1906 earthquake. In fact, Lota's fountain, which provided water to fight the fires that followed the earthquake, was located immediately in front of the building, which is now a Ritz Carlton property. For the next 15 years, this would be home for our medical group. No other doctors leased space in the building, just small businesses that included attorneys, accountants, and other professions that had nothing to do with medicine. I felt free.

150

There was always a sense of hustle-bustle at street level during business hours. Workers arrived between 8 and 9 a.m. via MUNI or BART, as parking in the Financial District was scarce and pricey. Throughout the day, bike messengers scurried about like kamikazes. It can be terrifying as a pedestrian or a driver to confront these demons, going the wrong way down one-way streets while transporting documents. Lunch hour brought the crowds out. Delis and food carts competed with some of the city's most elegant restaurants. Around 5 p.m., the commuters started to abandon the office buildings. After 6, the area resembled a ghost town.

Having real office space allowed us to build the business. Consulting rooms for mental health practitioners meant I had to find and hire those clinicians. Just as crucial, we needed office equipment and the professional staff to support the doctors. I don't take janitors for granted, and that also goes for administrative staff. Jane, my first administrative assistant, worked for a time in an office located in my home on Potrero Hill. There she kept records of appointments, produced consultative reports, and dealt with billing issues. It was a basic small-office operation.

Things were so much more efficient once we moved to Market Street and had all clinical and administrative functions in one location. Colleen was hired to work full time as an administrative assistant in the Market Street offices. To compete for competent staff with major businesses, we had to pay well, provide benefits, and have some perks. From early on, we had an old-style pension plan for employees who worked at least half time. We tried to be flexible about scheduling, a feature often desired by younger workers still pursuing college or graduate education.

I became sold on hiring employees who were smart and enthusiastic. We began requiring prospective employees for administrative jobs to complete testing during the screening process. If we expected examinees for clinical consultation to take a screening measure of intelligence, why not do so for potential hires? It's nice to employ smart folks. A 100-word spelling test was required as well. There's a big difference in job performance between a candidate who scores 95% and another who can't break the 80% threshold. A timed keyboarding and transcription test helped eliminate those who interviewed well but would never be able to produce as required when deadlines mattered. Some might say these assessments were discriminatory. That may be, but they are not only legal but humane. Why hire people who can't do the work or be trained for the job?

At the Center, company events celebrated our successes. Holiday meals at great restaurants were common. We had an Easter brunch at the Sheraton Palace, where staff brought their children to spend time with a human-sized bunny. There were outings to the outrageous Beach Blanket Babylon, a cabaret show. Occasionally, we'd arrange for off-site company events, with staff staying at the same hotel. There was even a weekend at spring training for the Giants in Scottsdale, Arizona. The point was to acknowledge staff and say, "Thank you." Other doctors have asked over the years how it is that my business manages to hire such competent, loyal employees. My answer is to take your time, be careful about whom you pick, and pay people well. Also, monitor their probationary period! We instituted an ongoing formal evaluation process that acknowledged areas of proficiency and assisted in improving performance throughout a worker's tenure with the company. Don't forget to pay people well. Incentive bonuses are very gratifying for employees to receive. Practice saying, "Thank you." Reward those who volunteer. And again, pay people well.

Greg came to work for the Center after a career in the Air Force. There was no need for psychological testing to establish his personality style. Greg was obsessive, in a good way. He took over after Colleen literally moved on to live elsewhere. Greg was the first employee The Center had who relished doing collections. He took great pride in charming claim's examiners with his Southern drawl until they released the insurer's purse strings. He viewed it as a personal insult when a payer resisted paying what was due. In those instances, he was like a dog on a bone, relentless.

Greg helped plan the move to 1390 Market Street when we were priced out of our downtown space. Our new offices were in a mixed-use high-rise complex in the Civic Center area of San Francisco. The Center would spend another 15 years there before again relocating due to rising rents, a phenomenon well known about San Francisco. The actual move took place the week of 9/11 in 2001. It went forward like a military exercise. Greg had arranged for the mover and all necessary logistical support from the new landlord. Sam, a part-time employee, was the other star of the relocation. He had the technical expertise to have the office networked by spending a weekend pulling cables with a buddy. We were up and running at a time that the country was in shock. Perhaps the move served as a distraction from the painful events we were witnessing on the news.

Some years later Sam left the company with money vested in the pension plan. He let us manage it until he rolled it over into an IRA. Sam's the son of immigrant parents from South Korea. He was a good guy who knew the value of saving. My wife Kim and I were invited to his wedding reception where we were honored to be among the few non-Asians in attendance. A Baptist minister gave the blessing in Korean.

Kim likes to remind me that she found Wendy. My wife had been an employment lawyer. She used a search firm to find a new office manager when Greg moved with his life partner to the state of Washington. Wendy has been the perfect fit. Everyone who crosses Wendy's path is impressed with her professionalism. She's married to a firefighter who is a man's man. They are good working people who get the job done. I try

152

not to upset her with my political views. Wendy is also a bit compulsive. She gets to work early. She likes things organized. She makes sure those with whom we do business follow through on their commitments.

Sometimes the doctors at the Center take for granted the numerous steps required to produce a finished consultative report or collect its final payment. I appreciate Wendy, so much so that I told her I would consider giving up my left arm before I'd see her leave her long-term office manager position.

The Center again relocated in 2016, this time to Oakland City Center. Real estate in San Francisco has become prohibitively expensive for many small businesses. We have downsized and adapted. When people call in, they hear Wendy's voice and find themselves confident that things will be taken care of. I couldn't do what I do without her. I am not alone. It's been a team effort.

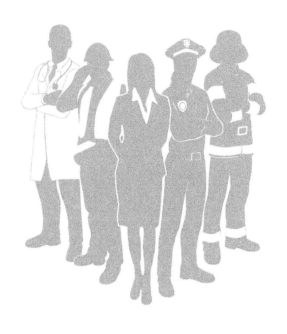

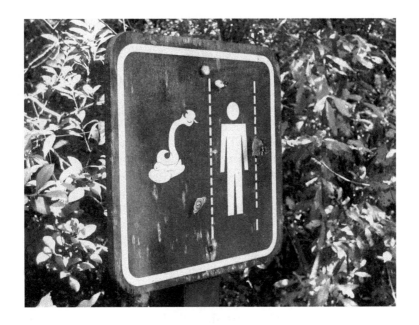

30 | Insurance Companies Are Not Our Friends

She was in her mid-30s when we met, a single woman referred by a colleague following her first psychiatric hospitalization. Grace had no history of psychiatric treatment before she ended up in an emergency room after an attempted overdose on alcohol and prescription drugs. She had been unhappy for some time, but her despair became like an avalanche after her most recent boyfriend broke up with her. She felt worthless. She projected into the future a lonely existence, where she would grow old in her studio apartment while continuing to work for a downtown employment agency that she did not believe in. She arrived on time for our first meeting, coming directly from work and dressed in a business suit. She brought the discharge medication prescribed by the psychiatrist responsible for her recent inpatient treatment.

Her doctor couldn't continue to oversee her care on an outpatient basis, but he had made sure Grace would receive needed follow-up from a psychiatrist, not just a master's level counselor. My colleague was concerned because the attempted suicide had been nearly successful. A neighbor with a key to Grace's small apartment was leaving a package for her when she found Grace unconscious on the floor. Rushed by ambulance to a nearby hospital, she had her stomach pumped and then stabilized after two days in an ICU. After being placed on an involuntary hold as a danger to self, Grace was transferred to a locked psychiatric unit where she found herself participating in individual counseling, going to group therapy with people she didn't know, and placed on an antidepressant for the first time in her life. No one visited her during her 10-day hospitalization.

Grace was embarrassed by the experience of nearly killing herself, ending up on a "psych ward," and having to take medication for depression. Back at work, she had concocted a story about her unexpected absence so co-workers might not discover she was so miserable. Over a period of four weeks, the medication seemed to be helping with her sleep, which had been disturbed for several months. She even regained her appetite and put on 5 pounds, which resulted in her looking healthier. Still quite sad in our sessions, she talked about her disappointments while agreeing that suicide was not the answer to what troubled her. She was becoming less at risk for a recurrence.

Then her employer's health insurance company denied authorization for the psychiatric services Grace was receiving. The initial billing was submitted after one month of treatment. My staff informed me that the problem had to do with my not being a member of the insurer's medical provider network, or "MPN." So, I took it upon myself to call the claims examiner assigned to Grace's case.

Dr. Bob:	"I received your bill review decision and was hoping to get clarification about the denial of authorization for treatment."
Insurance rep:	"OK. It's fairly simple, doctor. You're not a member of our panel of clinicians."
Dr. Bob:	"I assume your company covered my patient's hospitalization, both medical and psychiatric. Correct?"
Insurance rep:	"That's right. The inpatient treatment was found to be medically necessary, and so too would outpatient care with a designated provider."
Dr. Bob:	"Are you recommending that my patient begin again with a new doctor, when she's just becoming comfortable with her current psychiatrist?"

Insurance rep:	"Well, no. Her policy doesn't include coverage for her to meet with a psychiatrist."
Dr. Bob:	"What? This woman came very close to ending her life. She has only recently showed a positive response to medication. She has been diagnosed with a major depression that, if inadequately treated, could result in her ending up back in the hospital and on a disability leave!"
Insurance rep:	"Our mental health panel includes a number of good counselors."
Dr. Bob:	"Good counselors? Who will prescribe needed medication and monitor my patient's response?"
Insurance rep:	"She can go to her family doctor or her gynecologist. They're licensed physicians covered by her policy."
Dr. Bob:	"What if I accepted the same payment as the counselors on your MPN?"
Insurance rep:	"Doctor, she must meet with one of the master's level social workers or family therapists on the MPN for services to be reimbursed. Besides, the reimbursement is only $50."
Dr. Bob:	"Fine. I'll accept that as payment in full."
Insurance rep:	"That's not possible. She will have to go to an MPN counselor and a designated primary care doctor to receive coverage. I'm sorry."
Dr. Bob:	"You're sorry? Let me ask you a personal question. Do you and your family have this same lousy insurance?"
Insurance rep:	"Oh, no. I have what we refer to as Cadillac coverage that allows me to go to any board-certified psychiatrist. Of course, I don't see myself ever needing psychiatric care."
Dr. Bob:	"Right. If you reconsider your decision, please inform my office."

It took many weeks for me to help Grace find a competent psychotherapist acceptable to her insurer. I conferred with her primary care physician, who agreed with the need to maintain the antidepressant for some time. At our last session, my patient was considering changing her insurance coverage during her company's open enrollment period. She had met with her new therapist and had an appointment with her doctor. She thanked me for my services during her post-hospitalization recovery. I refused to take any payment, since she was already struggling financially. The Center wrote off the unpaid care as bad debt. I wished her well.

Some years later, I became a real patient when I developed a heart infection related to dental care. As I tell patients, "S*** happens." It took a while before my aortic valve began to fail as a result of the infection, and I eventually needed open heart surgery to replace the damaged valve. My surgeon prescribed a space-age form of treatment in anticipation of my surgery. I injected a "magic" protein into my abdomen for three weeks, which tricked my bone marrow into overproducing red blood cells. If the treatment worked, I might not require a blood transfusion during surgery and, as a result, would not be at risk for an infection such as hepatitis. My health insurance had authorized the hospitalization, the surgery, and my doctor's services. The insurer insisted that blood transfusions were reasonable, but not the injections to avoid them. When my surgeon's office had given up on receiving cooperation from the insurer, I called the utilization review nurse assigned to my pending claim.

Dr. Bob: "As a licensed physician, I'd like to explain the surgeon's rationale for prescribing the injections that are in dispute."

Nurse: "I have verified that you are a physician, and I see that you are even a member of the faculty at our local medical school. Please proceed."

Dr. Bob: "My surgeon intends to replace my aortic valve in two weeks. I will lose blood during the procedure, probably enough blood that I would need a blood transfusion. Your company would normally cover the transfusion. The transfusion has a small risk of exposing me to viruses. The injections will boost my blood count before surgery and are expected to make a transfusion unnecessary. In that scenario, there will be no risk of infection."

Nurse: "That sounds reasonable."

Dr. Bob: "So, you'll authorize the injection?"

Nurse: "No. You're the patient. We need to hear from your doctor's office."

Dr. Bob: "You know I'm a doctor, but you insist on calling my surgeon's office where you will speak to a secretary. My doctor is the busiest valve surgeon on the West Coast. He is either in surgery or driving home in his Ferrari to see his lovely wife. He does not spend time chatting with insurance company employees. His office staff won't be able to explain what the injections accomplish, and you probably won't be the one calling."

Nurse: "Doctor, that's how it works. Can I help you with anything else? I hope the surgery goes well."

That night I went home furious. Now I knew what my patients experienced when dealing with an insurer at odds with the treating physician's recommendations. I decided to pay several thousand dollars out of pocket for the injections and focused instead on taking care of the appointments in my office and entering the hospital with a positive state of mind. I awoke in the Cardiac Care Unit following surgery with a sense of joy for being alive. I required no transfusion due to my elevated blood count. I was fortunate that I was able to afford the out-of-pocket costs that many cannot. Four days after the successful surgery I was discharged.

While recuperating at home, I received a letter from the medical director of my health insurer stating that he had reviewed my claim and concluded that the injections, which had worked, were "experimental." That doctor never met with me. He is neither a heart surgeon nor an infectious disease expert. His judgment disregarded my surgeon having published the injection protocol in a peer-reviewed medical journal 13 years earlier. I was informed that I could appeal the denial of insurance coverage. I threw the doctor's letter in the trash.

I do not invest in insurance company stocks. I tried that briefly years ago and became disillusioned by the quarterly reports that focused on covered lives and profits used to purchase real estate. Don't get me wrong. I am not opposed to the concept of insurance, as it reduces risk should an untoward event take place. In my personal life and for my business, I carry multiple lines of insurance covering a range of potential disasters. I consider insurance to be a necessary evil, and my goal is to finish life having filed as few claims as possible. Insurers like it when we send them the checks and not vice versa. Not uncommonly, the fine print excludes coverage. If the claim is paid, premiums often go up or the insured no longer qualifies for future coverage. It's just my opinion, but insurance companies are not our friends.

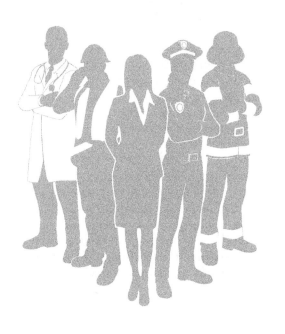

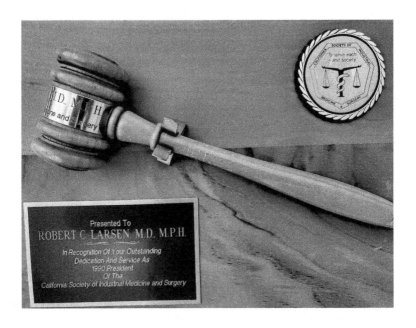

31 | Who Will Be Your Advocate?

Most people find no joy in the process of estate planning. Composing a last will and testament requires an individual to confront mortality. Avoidance and denial are powerful forces that argue for putting off decisions about what happens after we're gone. Aside from selecting a trustee to manage matters and deciding which potential beneficiaries should get which assets, there is usually a need to designate who has power of attorney to make health care decisions when we are unable to do so. The legal directive designates a trusted family member, friend, or colleague to make decisions regarding clinical intervention, including end-of-life options. That person becomes our advocate when we are incapable of choosing for ourselves.

In the course of studying public health and public policy, I was frequently exposed to the concept of health care advocacy. We can consider advocacy for the individual or the collective. The person who has your health care power of attorney advocates for you individually. Those who lobby for universal healthcare emphasize access to and coverage of quality treatment as fundamental rights for all, similar to clean air, clean water, and a safe supply of prescription drugs. All rights are limited, but in modern America, we continue to disagree about whether our fellow citizens have the right to decent medical care, or if it should be earned. Non-profit professional and lay associations make the case for universal healthcare coverage, while the argument against such invariably focuses on cost. Perhaps in the future, when basic health services are provided to all Americans, these old arguments will seem as antiquated as debates over the right to public education for all children, irrespective of family socioeconomics.

The Affordable Care Act (ACA) brought millions of Americans under the health insurance umbrella. Before the ACA, many working people could not afford to consult a physician about a suspicious cough or a breast lump. Families without health insurance could not risk injury, which commonly led to children of low-income households being excluded from playing sports. Young women without access to Planned Parenthood went without regular pap smears and oral contraception, which increased their chances of delayed cancer detection or of an unwanted pregnancy. The personal misery for the uninsured and the underinsured is immeasurable. The primary cause of personal bankruptcy in our country is related to health care costs, almost invariably due to inadequate insurance coverage. The ACA is likely the most notable public policy change for working-class Americans since the provision of Social Security, Medicare, and Medicaid benefits.

As a physician with additional training in public health and health policy, I believe doctors have a responsibility to advocate for a health-care system that covers all Americans. Is it not absurd that prisoners are guaranteed a right to health care in the United States, while working men and women are not? All too often, employed Americans are one paycheck away from financial disaster. In my practice, I routinely hear sagas from workers with admitted industrial injuries who have become destitute. While being treated for a back injury related to duties as a construction laborer, an employee may lose his job and with it, health insurance. Coverage of treatment for the work-related orthopedic problem and temporary disability benefits do not sufficiently make up for the financial burden of being without regular health insurance.

If the worker's employer is large enough, COBRA coverage might be available, but often at a cost that is unaffordable to someone struggling to get by on disability benefits. That same injured worker might no longer have prescription drug coverage for non-industrial health problems such as diabetes, hypertension, and hyperlipidemia. Once again, if the employee lives in a state participating in the ACA, then a safety net might be present. Without it, bankruptcy looms. The COVID-19 pandemic has highlighted issues of unemployment benefits and health insurance for Americans out of work.

When we consider the personal costs of bankruptcy following a serious illness or injury, we should also consider the adverse impact on the worker's self-esteem. No one wants to end up receiving Social Security benefits and going to the local food bank due to a prolonged recovery from a workplace tragedy. Such workers become depressed. They feel abandoned by their employer and the larger society. They routinely battle with their employer's workers' compensation carrier over disability benefits and authorization for recommended treatment. With time, they become worn down and see themselves as useless and of little value. They might abuse their pain medication and increase their intake of alcohol to self-medicate the chronic physical and emotional pain. Their ties to productive, working friends become fragile, and they begin to identify with the disabled population. The risk for suicide rises.

~~~~~~

I am reminded of the resilience of a former sex worker in San Francisco. Sarah came to the Bay Area after graduating from college with a degree in liberal arts. She worked in restaurants where she made enough to support herself while living in a shared rental apartment with other young adult women. During an economic downturn, the restaurant where she worked as a bartender closed after losing its lease. Sarah collected unemployment benefits and barely got by during a job search, which did not pan out. Another blow came when she was evicted after the building, where she had lived for several years, was sold. Sarah ended up homeless. Friends gave her temporary shelter. By this time, she had given up on finding work and started hanging out at a bar, leading to increased alcohol use. One of the guys at the bar shared some of his cocaine with her. It improved her mood, at least temporarily.

Sarah's use of illicit substances transitioned to the cheaper drug methamphetamine, which she could barter for with sexual favors from her connection. Intravenous drug use followed, and her life continued on a downhill spiral. The friends who provided housing kicked her out and pleaded with the former bartender to "get your s*** together." Sarah became a sex worker on the streets of the Tenderloin district of San Francisco, providing her services in exchange for money, drugs, or a place to crash. For the first time in her life, she ended up in the criminal justice system. Her crimes were non-violent and involved prostitution and drug possession. During one of her times in the county jail, she got clean and sober. Sarah was befriended by a social worker who got her into a halfway house for women in recovery.

The former sex worker learned of an innovative program sponsored by Coyote, the sex workers' union. Only in San Francisco would a former prostitute and recovering drug addict be seen as a good prospective employee. Her new job was as a public health educator to sex workers. Sarah got along well with poor women who walked the streets of the city. She knew a number of them from her working days. As a sex worker educator, she emphasized the use of condoms and clean needles with her clientele. The job required Sarah to demonstrate how to place a condom on an erect penis during oral sex. For demonstration purposes, she made use of a banana. Nevertheless, her sponsor in a 12-step program thought the new job was too risky for someone at Sarah's early stage of recovery.

It took several months as a sex worker educator before Sarah once again started to deteriorate. It began when she was arrested by rookie cops who would not accept her identification card as a Public Health Department employee. Then, after being assaulted by a John looking for sex, she ended up being treated for multiple soft tissue injuries at San Francisco General. She returned to the bar she had been avoiding and resumed her use of IV drugs, attempting to treat her physical pain and emotional suffering.

To support her renewed drug habit, Sarah once again became a sex worker. She was discharged from the halfway house for breaking her sobriety, resulting in her again living on the dangerous streets of the Tenderloin. The pattern of repeat incarceration resumed. Sarah was approached by the same social worker who had helped her in the past. This time, she suggested that Sarah file a workers' compensation claim for cumulative injury resulting from a job that placed her in a high-risk environment for a recovering addict.

Sarah got legal counsel and prevailed when her claim was found to be compensable. Since her claim predated changes to California's workers' comp system, she was awarded extensive vocational rehabilitation benefits. She enrolled at San Francisco State University and obtained a Master's Degree in Public Policy. During her graduate studies, she maintained her sobriety. She could also afford a studio apartment with her modest disability benefits.

When she was evaluated in our offices, Sarah's case was about to be settled. My report chronicled the good and bad behavior she exhibited since losing the restaurant position and her apartment some years ago. She presented as a fashionably attired 40-year-old woman who was articulate about many provocative tales. Her goal was clear, to maintain her progress while being of service to others. She had recently interviewed for a job in the San Francisco Department of Public Health. She was optimistic that she was a good candidate for the position, which involved working with various agencies as an advocate for marginalized women with histories of abuse, who not uncommonly resorted to selling their bodies to get by.

This prospective job would require Sarah to work with the police, the courts, the county hospital and clinics, homeless shelters, and recovery programs while representing vulnerable persons like she had been. She was stronger now, and there was an obvious purpose to her mission to help others escape a life of tragic desperation. More than a year later, I read a story about Sarah in the San Francisco Chronicle. She was being recognized for her advocacy in representing the forgotten women of the Tenderloin and demonstrating by example that they too could have a future.

The story of an individual who has lost everything and comes back from the abyss should leave us with hope. Hope that connects us to something greater than ourselves. Hope that brings renewal from despair. Sarah's is a story of resilience in a worker who, importantly, had an advocate. We have not survived as a species without such hardiness and mutual support.

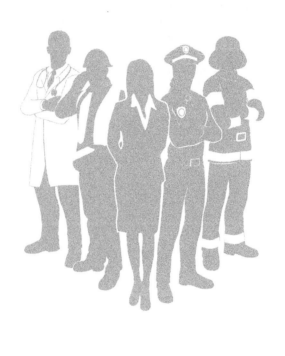

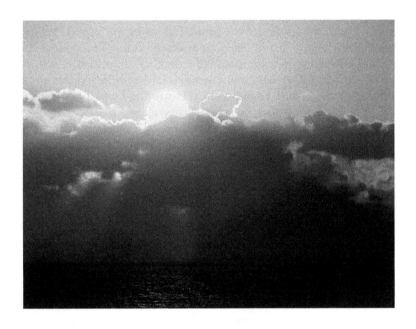

32 | The Value of Psychotherapy

I **come from a background that emphasized science and** the importance of evidence. Cell biologists explore the mystery of life through techniques such as electron microscopic imagery and gel electrophoresis. I have always been attracted to dramatic photographs that capture some truth about existence. This is true of historical images of war, portraits of the famous and infamous, broad landscape shots in color as well as black and white, and the imagery of the elegant universe of the intracellular environment. Who would have predicted that this medical student, functioning as a teaching assistant to his peers learning microbiology, would go on to pursue a career in the squishy field of medicine known as psychiatry?

My psychiatric training came at a time when "biological" psychiatry was gaining strength. Greater attention was being given to neurotransmitters and drugs designed to impact on receptor sites of neurons. One would think it was the perfect time for a biologist to become impressed with the science of the brain and mind, and it was. Yet it was also a point when the art of listening and responding to a patient made sense as well. To complicate matters further, while trained in science, I grew up with a mother who was superstitious and believed that dreams could foretell the future. Fortunately, the training I was lucky to receive at UCSF did not minimize the value of psychology. Residents in psychiatry were expected to engage in psychotherapy with our patients, just as were trainees in psychology. It was never all about addressing symptoms and complaints through prescribing a cocktail of drugs.

During my four years of residency training, I sought out my own psychotherapy or analysis. The justification for that process was that it would assist me to better understand which were my issues and, therefore, not those of my patients. As a scientist, I liked the romantic notion that I would be the instrument to assess my patient's state of mind and to measure the response to treatment. In the midst of my Jungian analysis, I learned that I was a sensation type. That explained my appreciation for the visual arts, spicy food, and music.

My lengthy process of individual psychotherapy with Dr. Peter Rutter forced me to engage in self-reflection. My analyst once told me he thought of me when seeing a vehicle with the vanity license plate: ALL NOW. That took a while to sink in. Yes, that captured this ambitious first-generation American in Dr. Rutter's office. I would have to come to grips with my compulsive traits and competitive drives, both of which had been reinforced by growing up in an upwardly mobile family and an educational system that rewarded "honors" performance.

Apart from my own experience in therapy, which I lightly refer to as incomplete, there is the cumulative work as therapist to others, which is humbling for the honest clinician. Change takes time and patience. Taking on the role of patient in psychotherapy, aspiring doctors learn empathy, if they are fortunate. As instructive as it is to suffer physical illness or injury for physicians to understand what our patients feel, so too is it crucial for doctors to grapple with their own demons to encourage patients to also do so. In retrospect, my participation in therapy was not all about refining my instrument, as it also helped me to grow up and be a better person, both within and outside of the professional setting.

It would be incorrect to conclude that psychotherapy is the "art" of psychiatry, while medication management represents the "science" of that field. Psychotherapy works through a series of human interactions that incrementally change the brain at the molecular, cellular, and structural levels. Emotions are touched upon. Memories are revisited. Relationships are explored. Accompanying alterations in coping, self-image, and social ties involve RNA (ribonucleic acid) and protein synthesis. In such cases, nerve pathways can be altered.

The Decade of the Brain spanned the years of 1990 through 1999, with continued major advancements in neuroscience. However, our appreciation for the value of psychotherapy did not lessen. In fact, numerous studies found that where medication is beneficial in addressing symptoms of depression and anxiety, psychotherapy adds further benefit. We were starting to understand the effect of psychotherapy. If fear and anxiety emanate from the primitive portion of the brain known as the limbic system, then we believe the overriding control is centered in the prefrontal cortex. Cognitive behavioral therapy is effective in treating anxiety and depression. It works by changing our assessments of situations and strengthening coping skills. Essentially, the patient learns to respond in a more adaptive manner to cues that, in the past, brought forth fear and sadness. Perhaps the prefrontal cortex of the brain inhibits the action of the more deeply located amygdala, from which anxiety symptoms are generated.

Research to date underscores the value of psychotherapy to assist the patient in developing better coping skills. Unlike pharmacotherapy and other biologic forms of treatment, such as electroconvulsive therapy, psychotherapy has few adverse effects. Furthermore, the benefits achieved via psychotherapy need not end when treatment does. We actually can become a "better me." Just as surgery might be one component of treatment of physical illness and disease, it does not mitigate the use of drugs or lifestyle changes. So too can psychotherapy and pharmacotherapy be seen as complementary in the treatment of mental disorders. These synergistic effects of treatment will continue to grow as we study early-childhood development, brain trauma, genomics, cognitive functioning, and the various states of mind the human species experiences.

In a world that emphasizes multi-tasking, should there not be a balance struck with treatment mechanisms that instead require contemplation? Psychotherapy and counseling services in general focus on the self in a social existence. They are exercise for the psyche. Though some see such services as self-indulgent, they can be life-saving. Psychotherapy, however, takes more effort than downing a pill twice a day. The same can be said for regular physical exercise compared to taking a drug to address diabetes or high blood pressure. The take-home message is that coming to a better awareness of one's self can make a positive difference in how we function and relate to those around us. With that improved functioning comes a reduction in symptoms and complaints. That is the value of psychotherapy.

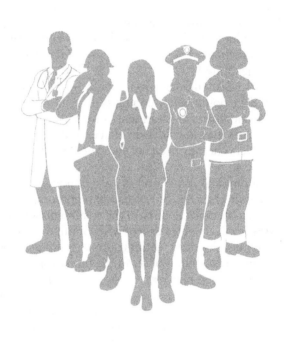

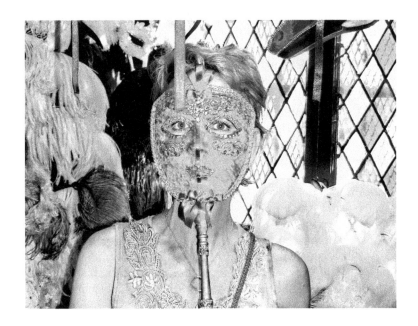

33 | Lulus

In medical school, we referred to the most curious cases as "fascinomas," for their fascinating nature. That's a designation no one wants to be labeled with, for good reason. Anytime you find yourself in a teaching hospital and the professor makes a point of bringing all the trainees to your bedside, it's not because you're a delightful conversationalist. You likely have an unusual clinical presentation. In psychiatry, the bizarre cases can be designated as "lulus."

A male office worker in his early 30s was scheduled for an evaluation in our offices related to his claim of job stress. I was organizing the copious records when the claimant, Mr. Green, showed up a couple of days early for his appointment. He requested that he be allowed to photograph me with his records. He believed that by chronicling me in the presence of many volumes of medical and administrative records, he would assure his records would be safeguarded from persons intending to steal them before they were returned to his attorney's office. I agreed with the request and stood behind the documents, which were neatly stacked on my desk.

I didn't comment that the stacks of paper, bound volumes of records, and deposition transcripts were not identifiable as Mr. Green's records, based upon the camera images. He then asked me to pose with his invention, which others had allegedly been interested in acquiring. It was a disc brake system for skateboards. I held the skateboard so the sign on the bottom of its deck could be read. It stated, "The braking system for this skateboard is the property of I. M. Green. Its design is covered by a pending patent registered to Mr. Green. Any use of this design or copying of it is strictly prohibited."

Two days later, Mr. Green arrived for his appointment and fully cooperated in completing a battery of psychological testing before our interview. By then, I had gone through his records, which told a tale of mistrust and interpersonal sensitivity that was hard to fathom. He had grown up in an intact family where both of his parents were immigrants. He was the oldest of three sons. His parents worked in restaurants while he grew up in the Bay Area. In public schools, he did well in math and science classes. He did not date as a teenager because his parents were reportedly very strict. After graduating from high school, he studied computer science at the local community college. After three years, he completed the requirements for his associate's degree.

During his college years, Mr. Green continued living in the family home, while supporting himself as a computer tech for a small shop in the neighborhood. He enrolled at a state university, then changed his major from computer technology to mechanical engineering, after an argument with a computer science professor over a grade on a mid-term exam. Mr. Green filed a discrimination complaint with the university, claiming the professor had altered his answers on the test. An investigation failed to support the allegations, and it was suggested that the student get counseling through the student health service on campus. That never happened.

Mr. Green took three more years to obtain his B.S. in engineering. During that time, he avoided taking more computer classes because he was convinced that the professors in that department intended to punish him for making a formal complaint. He quit his job as a computer tech after he learned that his boss was providing networking services to the computer science department at his university. He could no longer trust that employer, who he believed was secretly communicating with the professor who had cheated him. Mr. Green then found a job working for a skateboard shop in the Haight Ashbury district of the city. This became his dream job, for a time. He loved tinkering in the parts department during his breaks. He became so adept at repairing skateboards that within three months, he was promoted to lead repair technician.

Mr. Green's work at the skateboard shop ended when he became convinced that the owner was planning to take credit for his invention. The owner had become aware of the disc brake system that his employees were testing for their co-worker. He complimented Mr. Green on his ingenuity but commented that such a braking system was both impractical and too expensive to be used by skateboarders. Concerned that the owner would acquire the rights to his invention if he remained an employee, he quit. Mr. Green was then hired by an engineering firm as a drafter. He accepted the job offer only after receiving assurance that any invention of his that predated his hire would be of no interest to the prospective employer.

Mr. Green finished his probationary employment without difficulty. He was technically proficient and demonstrated a positive attitude through his attendance and volunteering for overtime projects. His employer suggested that he spend more time with co-workers during their breaks. At the company holiday party, Mr. Green showed up with his skateboard and prototype braking system. He encouraged his peer group to try it out, and they took him up on his offer. This resulted in a co-worker going to a local emergency room for treatment of a fractured left forearm. The following week, Mr. Green met with his department manager, who indicated that he showed poor judgment in bringing his invention to a company event. The manager made it clear that the business did not need any more injury claims.

Not long after the company party, Mr. Green overheard two technicians talking about a patent that the firm was hoping to acquire for mountain bikes. It was for brakes that were lightweight and used a disc design! Oh my, the assurance from the human resources (HR) department that his invention would remain his property had been a ruse. Mr. Green went to his manager, accusing the company of pilfering his ideas. The manager denied having any knowledge of a plot to defraud the employee and promised Mr. Green that he'd look into the situation.

The next day, the manager met with Mr. Green and an HR representative to explain to the employee that the bicycle brakes had been planned for two years, predating his hire. The manager brought in a prototype and demonstrated how its mechanics and materials were unlike the skateboard brake. The HR representative stated that Mr. Green's invention was not something the company had any interest in, and it was hoped he would be successful in fulfilling his dream.

The meeting ended when Mr. Green began hyperventilating and collapsed to the floor while getting up from his chair. He struck his head and was briefly unconscious. Paramedics arrived after the manager called 911. At the local ER, he was diagnosed with a closed head injury and a post-concussion syndrome. While off work for his physical injuries, Mr. Green obtained legal counsel for his workers' compensation claim, which was amended to include cumulative stress. He also consulted with labor law attorneys in an attempt to stop his employer from producing the bicycle brakes, which he still contended were based upon his design.

Mr. Green was getting by on temporary disability benefits. His treating doctor had recommended he consult with a psychologist, given his conviction that his employer was plotting against him. The physical medicine doctor assigned to the case was not interested in being photographed with his patient's invention. Mr. Green's deposition was taken by the employer's attorney, given the claim that the company was involved in nefarious activities directed toward using the employee's invention without permission. Meanwhile, Mr. Green's physical injuries were found to be modest and would not prevent him from resuming his draftsman duties.

Neither the employer nor the employee was interested in continuing Mr. Green's employment with the engineering company. Mr. Green, while describing himself as perturbed by the company's actions, did not see himself as needing psychiatric care. His psychological test results were consistent with an individual of high average intelligence who did not come across as depressed or anxious yet was concerned about his physical health and mistrustful to the point of endorsing symptoms of paranoia. My opinion was that Mr. Green had a pre-existing mental disorder, i.e., a delusional disorder, which manifested itself in the work setting. The workplace had acted as a passive stage for playing out his psychopathology. His case was later settled. I learned that Mr. Green continued living in his parents' home while his younger siblings had become independent. He was still in search of investors for his invention.

ৎৡৢ৶ৡৢ৶ৡৢ৶ৡৢ৶ৡৢ৶ৡৢ৶ৡৢ৶ৡৢ৶ৡৢ৶ৡৢ৶ৡৢ৶ৡ

The case of Ms. Chun raises the concept that, for some people, an injury can bring on an unexpected response. She was seen in our offices four years after experiencing an acute low back strain while working as a clinic nurse. Now at the age of 50, she was intending to apply for Social Security benefits based upon combined physical and mental disability. The primary injury was to the low back, and an MRI scan demonstrated two bulging discs for which surgery was not recommended. Ms. Chun had ended physical therapy because she was convinced it had made her pain worse. She had been receiving regular chiropractic adjustments, but there was no indication they had improved her functioning.

In addition to unrelenting back pain, Ms. Chun complained of neck pain, upper extremity weakness, headaches, dizziness, and urinary incontinence. She claimed that her tongue uncontrollably protruded to the

174

right side. She also noticed that since the lifting injury, she had begun to experience seasonal allergies for the first time in her life. Her doctors recommended she meet with a psychologist. She enjoyed meeting with that mental health practitioner and having someone who would listen to her in the midst of her continued deterioration.

The medical workup was extensive but, other than the MRI scan results, did not demonstrate any significant objective pathology. There was no explanation for Ms. Chun's neck pain, headaches, and weakness. Electrical studies of the nerves in her upper extremities were unimpressive. Scans of the brain and cervical spine likewise demonstrated no significant abnormality. A consulting neurologist found give-way weakness most consistent with a psychosomatic presentation, apart from the admitted back strain. Testing of Ms. Chun's bladder function gave no indication that there was a physical basis for the reported incontinence.

An evaluating orthopedist concluded that Ms. Chun had a legitimate, though minor, back disability. A "global pain syndrome" was thought to have prominent psychological underpinnings. After meeting with Ms. Chun, who cried and appeared to be in excruciating pain during the interview, I consulted with the orthopedist. He reiterated his findings and concluded by stating, "I have no idea why this nice lady has become a cripple. I think she's a Lulu. You're the shrink. You make sense of it."

At times, profound psychosomatic illness can arise for reasons that make sense. For many individuals, physical complaints are considered more legitimate than reporting features of emotional distress. Persons with histrionic personality characteristics are at increased risk for putting forth unfounded physical symptoms. Patients with histories of abuse are also prone toward becoming passive and dependent in response to a relatively minor event. None of these factors explained what was taking place with Ms. Chun. Her medical history did not show her to have had any pre-existing hypochondriacal tendencies. Her family life was stable. She had no past psychiatric treatment.

Ultimately, Ms. Chun's claims were resolved. She received some continued care for her back with the expectation that surgery would not be pursued. At least in that regard, no further harm would take place from an aggressive surgeon and a willing healthcare system. She continued to make use of various herbs and supplements. An antidepressant was instituted to address mood, pain, and sleep difficulties. She remained a broken person with numerous pain and other subjective complaints of unknown origin. There was no miracle.

სიტყ სიტყ სიტყ სიტყ სიტყ სიტყ სიტყ სიტყ სიტყ სიტყ

At times, a person presents with a story that appears implausible. Such was the case of Mr. Johnson, a middle-aged garbage man. He had been a long-term employee of a waste management company, and for years had worked on a truck collecting trash. Later, he bid for a position at the employer's solid waste disposal site that involved separating recyclables from general waste to be buried in a landfill. Mr. Johnson had a reputation as a responsible worker who would work extra shifts when the need arose. His last assignment was at the company's new recycling yard, where his duties involved accepting recyclables such as glass, plastic, and cardboard from the public. He also had regular dealings with co-workers who transported bins of recyclables from other sites. His location did not accept electronics or toxic liquids such as paint and chemicals, so he tried to be of service by referring customers with those items to the appropriate disposal sites.

Not long after coming to the recycling yard, Mr. Johnson found himself at odds with some of the staff there. He went to the general manager after being subjected to racial slurs by two cousins who worked the night shift. It was his word against the cousins, as there were no other witnesses. One day at lunch, Mr. Johnson noticed a foul odor coming from the paper bag his meal was in. He asked others in the lunchroom whether someone might have tampered with his food. Hearing only denials, he took a bite from the sandwich his wife had prepared. A bitter taste caused him to spit the food out. He heard a snicker or two. After throwing out the sandwich, he found his immediate supervisor, who assured him his concerns would be investigated. Three days later, an HR manager from headquarters met with Mr. Johnson to report that interviews of co-workers had found no wrongdoing. If something similar happened again, he should save the evidence and not discard it.

Back at the lunchroom that day, a table of co-workers got up and left as Mr. Johnson entered the room. He ate his meal but afterwards found himself experiencing abdominal cramping and diarrhea and went home early. The next day, he still felt nauseous and called in sick. He returned to work the following day after consulting with a union representative. The employee put the employer on notice that he wished to submit a claim for physical injury as a result of being poisoned and an additional claim for job stress. His regular physician placed him on a leave of absence. His union referred him to an attorney, who arranged for medical and psychiatric evaluations.

Not surprisingly, the medical evaluation was inconclusive as to whether Mr. Johnson had been poisoned. The evaluating physician concluded that it was as likely that he had experienced an episode of acute gastroenteritis as it was that his food had been tainted by others at the worksite. Mr. Johnson presented in my office as irritable while insisting that someone needed to protect him from the bigots at his workplace who had it out for him. His psychological test results were consistent with an individual who was angry, mistrustful, and worried about his health. His personnel file demonstrated that he had been an employee with no serious performance problems before he worked at the recycling center.

An investigation conducted by the employer's insurer found no corroboration for Mr. Johnson's allegations. Interviews of co-workers described him as someone who kept to himself without making an effort to become part of the team. Having not much else to go by, my psychiatric report could not conclude that his problems were work-related. I recommended that the employer negotiate a transfer back to Mr. Johnson's prior assignment. If additional evidence surfaced, I was interested in considering it, because the available data were insufficient to render an opinion about what had caused this previously reliable employee to make such outlandish claims.

While it might appear that Mr. Johnson's presentation could be ascribed to the machinations of a Lulu, that turned out not to be the case. Two months after I submitted my report, I received a request to reconsider my opinions based upon new information pertinent to the case. A former office employee had learned that Mr. Johnson was on a leave from work. This woman had worked in a trailer at the recycling center while Mr. Johnson was employed there. She had submitted a sworn affidavit that she had heard two workers laughing about putting a laxative in Mr. Johnson's food. Some derogatory comments about his race were also made at the time.

The office worker had not reported what she had overheard, because those employees had previously harassed a different worker, who quit out of frustration. The office worker was concerned about potential retaliation. She had transferred back to headquarters while Mr. Johnson was on a leave of absence. The new information she provided changed everything. Now the claimant's physical and mental problems were accepted as compensable. The responsible employees were terminated, and Mr. Johnson returned to the recycling yard, where he was no longer considered to be a problem.

൞ ൞ ൞ ൞ ൞ ൞ ൞ ൞ ൞ ൞ ൞ ൞ ൞

Facts make a difference in occupational medicine, especially in unusual cases. Sometimes it can take years to establish what causal factors are involved in bringing about illness in an individual worker or even in a group of employees. At times, the easy solution is to conclude that the worker is crazy or a Lulu whose account cannot be believed.

Following the Gulf War in Kuwait, a number of U.S. military members filed claims that involved a variety of physical and emotional symptoms. Initially, those claims were considered to be some type of psychological reaction to combat. However, it turned out that those soldiers had been exposed to low-level uranium used in artillery to strengthen projectiles. These were cases of toxic exposure and not PTSD. Before concluding that a tale that is difficult to understand is coming from a Lulu, I always have to make sure there is not some other plausible explanation.

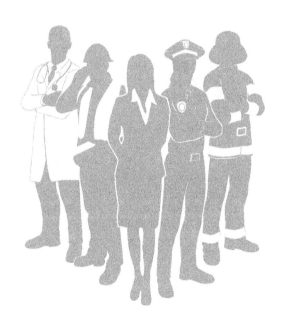

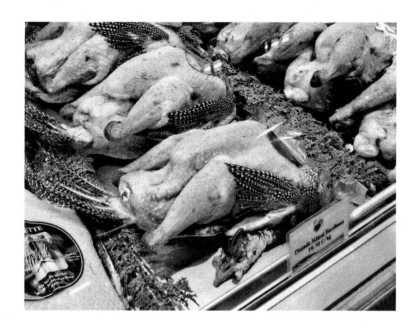

34 | Job Title: Killer

When looking through an employee's personnel
file, it is common to find a written job description. Job
descriptions help applicants learn about requirements
as well as the duties inherent to a given job. Doctors
might be asked to review a job description when releasing a patient
back to regular duty following a medical leave of absence. State and
federal laws might also require a physician offering an opinion about
a worker's ability to perform a particular job to consult the essential
and non-essential duties detailed in a job description. Per the Americans
with Disabilities Act (ADA), a person who can perform the essential job
functions, with or without reasonable accommodation, is protected.

ॐ◈ॐ◈ॐ◈ॐ◈ॐ◈ॐ◈ॐ◈ॐ◈ॐ◈ॐ◈ॐ◈ॐ◈ॐ◈ॐ◈ॐ◈

Ms. Kumar was an immigrant in her early 50s when referred to our offices for evaluation of her state of mind. She and her family had emigrated from her homeland of India more than a decade before we met. The Kumar family came to California, where they resided in the same community as her brother-in-law. So many immigrants had come to the Central Valley of California that a city there is named Delhi, though pronounced differently than the one in India.

For years, Ms. Kumar raised her three children in India while her husband labored on farms in California. She and her children were later reunited with their father in Merced County. When the youngest child had completed high school, Ms. Kumar decided to begin working outside of the family home. She had grown up in a village in India where her father was a farmer. Her marriage to her husband had been arranged by both families. She spoke respectfully about her husband as a man who worked hard, provided for his family, and loved his children. Her interest in finding employment came from a desire to help out with expenses and to reduce the burden on her spouse.

A large poultry processing center employing more than 5,000 workers was located in the area where Ms. Kumar lived. Many of the plant workers were immigrants like Ms. Kumar. In fact, there were so many immigrants at that worksite that she learned she would receive instructions in her native dialect, as well as in English. With only a modest formal education in her homeland and none in this country, Ms. Kumar was hired with no prior job experience. The title of her job position was "Killer."

The written job description was for an entry-level position where the employee would work 10 hours per shift, four shifts per week. Protective clothing, including zippered white coveralls with a hood, high-top rubber boots, gloves, and goggles, would be provided. She would be assigned to a work station where she would stand in a slurry of chicken feathers and blood. Approximately 100,000 chickens would pass by, hanging from their feet on an overhead conveyor belt, in a single work shift. A din of machinery and chicken cackles saturated the air. The Killer's primary task was to cut the throat of any chicken that survived the machinery that provided an intended lethal electric shock. This action had to be performed with precision while the birds sped by the work station.

I was both impressed with and horrified by this employee's job description, which I read before our meeting. She had worked at the job for many months before she was injured. There were no adverse job actions in her file. She had done what was asked of her until the day she lost a thumb. Ms. Kumar recalled reaching up to cut the throat of a chicken that was flailing about. She made the fatal cut as she had done on many other occasions. This time, the struggle with the bird lasted long enough for the glove on her right hand to catch on a conveyor hook. She instinctively pulled back as the machine forcefully amputated her thumb. Co-workers heard her screams and came to her aid. The line was shut down, but the thumb was never found. A clean towel was put on the wound while Ms. Kumar waited for emergency personnel to arrive.

Taken to a local trauma center, the worker's wound was irrigated, the bleeding stopped, and the hand sutured. Follow-up was arranged with a hand surgeon. She went home still wondering whether she might be experiencing a bad dream. But it was not, and she found herself revisiting the incident that cost her the thumb on her dominant hand. She was convinced that she could have done something to avoid this tragedy.

In the weeks that followed the amputation of her thumb, Ms. Kumar learned that only limited clinical intervention was possible. After swelling had lessened, a skilled hand surgeon addressed the damaged tissue and closed up the site. While transplantation of a big toe was proposed, the risks and potential poor outcome of that procedure were not attractive to Ms. Kumar. She was referred by the insurer to a physical medicine specialist for management of her pain. She was placed on an anticonvulsant to reduce the numbness and tingling. She also experienced phantom limb pain, as though the thumb were still present and being poked with a needle.

We met several months later, when Ms. Kumar had begun to understand the extent of her loss. While it involved only one digit on her hand, she felt as though she would never be whole. She had received physical therapy and learned to grasp with the affected hand or to use her left hand for certain tasks, but she still felt clumsy. She had been encouraged by doctors and her physical therapist not to hide her damaged extremity. She was aware that others at times stared at her "mangled" hand. She could no longer use that hand for forceful gripping and grasping or tasks involving fine dexterity. Because she could no longer perform the essential duties for her usual job as Killer, and no reasonable accommodation was possible, she lost her position, along with her thumb. No alternative position with the company had been offered. She felt abandoned.

In our meeting, Ms. Kumar came across as cooperative, reserved, and polite. With the assistance of an interpreter, she completed written test measures. She admitted feeling sad about the permanent injury to her hand and believed her prospects for the future were limited. At the same time, she felt supported by her family, who helped out with tasks that were now a challenge for her.

Ms. Kumar's case was ultimately settled after she had access to counseling and a trial of an antidepressant to address mood, pain, and sleep symptoms. Her disability award, which provided for both physical and mental injury, was modest, given the impact that her job at the poultry plant had on her life. Sometimes, there are no good answers or remedies for a worker who is seriously hurt because of doing her job.

In this case, all who provided service to Ms. Kumar wished that more could have been done to correct the wrong that had occurred. Her situation left us all feeling impotent.

◈◈◈◈◈◈◈◈◈◈◈◈◈◈◈◈◈◈◈◈◈◈◈

Jake, a man in his late 30s, was seen in our offices after injuring his low back. He had been employed by a rendering plant that disposed of dead cattle. His job struck me as being as gruesome as the Killer's. For about a dozen years, Jake had "been my own man," driving a route in California's Fresno County to pick up dead cows at dairy farms. His job involved using a mechanical winch to pull the body of the dead cow onto the bed of a truck. He then transported the animal to the plant, where other workers processed the remains. Many of the cows died while giving birth or simply from aging. When I remarked to Jake that his job sounded pretty awful, he responded, "Oh no, doc. I loved that job. I loved the smell of those farms. I loved seeing the healthy animals. I loved being out on those open roads. I miss it."

After he initially injured his back slipping in bodily fluids of a dead adult cow, Jake was sent for orthopedic consultation. He had developed bulging of a lumbar disc, which was impinging on nerve roots. Surgery was performed at one level of his spine in an effort to eliminate the disc bulging and the associated nerve impingement. The postoperative recovery was going as expected. The treating surgeon indicated that after several months, Jake could return to work at limited duty. The employer then assigned Jake to a route where he would handle only dead calves and not any full-grown bovine. The alternative duties lasted less than a month, when Jake was reinjured pulling on a length of chain used to haul in a dead calf.

The MRI scan demonstrated a herniated disc that was beyond repair. Jake had further surgery to remove the damaged disc and to install plating and screws, with the goal of fusing two vertebrae and stabilizing the spine. After more than a year, the surgeon concluded his patient had recovered as much as could be expected. The problem was that even with an acceptable surgical outcome, no heavy lifting was recommended. Jake no longer could perform his regular job, and his basic academic skills did not qualify him for a less strenuous job in the company's offices. His prospects for future employment were poor.

Jake arrived on time for his psychiatric evaluation at our office. He wasn't quite sure why others thought he needed to see a "shrink." He was going along with what was recommended, just as he had with so many other clinicians he had seen since his first injury. He made clear that he hoped no one saw him as "crazy." His gait was awkward, in part because he had developed a foot drop after the second injury and surgery. Jake had not done well in public schools, where he enjoyed

182

football and shop classes. He had a few entry-level jobs before landing the job hauling dead dairy cattle. A family member suggested he find an attorney after his employer notified him that he was being let go, because he could not return to his prior duties. It was his attorney who wanted assessment of his client's emotions.

Jake was not a complainer, although he missed many aspects of his job. He seemed relieved when told he had no major mental illness and that it was normal to be sad about how the injuries had changed his life. Other doctors said he probably would qualify for Social Security disability benefits. He instead intended to take a job as a parking lot attendant that did not involve any lifting. Jake's case was settled, acknowledging that he was left with some reduced self-confidence in addition to his various musculoskeletal impairments. Like Ms. Kumar, Jake could not be made whole. Unfortunately, those with legitimate injuries cannot always be put back together so their lives can go on as usual. Life as seen in these cases is not fair.

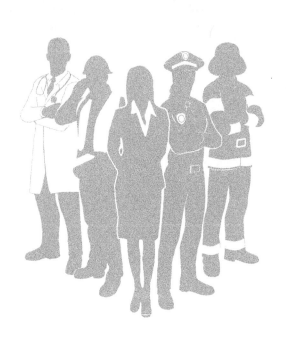

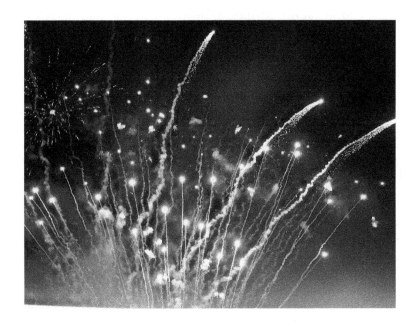

35 | Overcoming Victimization

Mind over matter is an ancient concept. It commonly has to do with willpower winning out over physical adversity. The impossible is possible. An object too heavy to lift is lifted. A shipwrecked sailor survives longer than imagined possible. A physician performs her own mastectomy while stationed in an isolated location of Antarctica. Humans ascend and summit Mount Everest without the use of supplemental oxygen. Herculean feats are achieved through determination. Might not the unexpected come forth in responding to trauma as well? Of course, it does.

Physicians tend to give attention to pathology. Our training emphasizes illness and disease rather than optimal health. Patients seek out medical intervention when they don't feel right. Doctors in turn conduct examinations to identify what's wrong more so than what's working fine. It makes sense. The same is true of psychiatry and psychology, which primarily focus on disturbances of mood, behavior, and thoughts, as opposed to giving attention to excellent coping and satisfying relationships. It's crucial to discover what can be fixed and not get caught up in what is functioning well.

It is important to realize that there are ranges across human behavior and emotions. Understandable mistrust is distantly related to paranoid delusions. Reasonable trepidation is on a continuum that ends in immobilizing anxiety. A period of grief following the loss of a loved one is distinct from suicidal depression. Why is it that not all those exposed to profound life-threatening trauma develop PTSD? Just as not all immune systems are equal, so it is that some individuals have more psychological immunity than others.

Many of my colleagues are fascinated by, conduct research upon, and prescribe treatment for patients with recognized PTSD and major depression. Should not those persons exposed to similar levels of trauma and loss, who persevere without becoming emotionally disturbed, deserve attention as well? While a just society recognizes disability and provides accommodations, imagine if we routinely rewarded resilience.

୬ଈ୬ଈ୬ଈ୬ଈ୬ଈ୬ଈ୬ଈ୬ଈ୬ଈ୬ଈ୬ଈ୬ଈ

Charles had last worked full time as a respiratory therapist 12 years before we met. The medical director for a major insurance company had suggested that I consult on his case. Two days after Charles had provided inhalation therapy to a patient with a pulmonary infection, he became symptomatic. He was on a fishing trip with a buddy when he found himself coughing, running a fever, and sweating through the night. He called his wife, who was a registered nurse. She advised that he get himself to an emergency room ASAP. The nurse knew that her husband treated some seriously ill patients at a major medical center. It turned out that Charles had provided care to a patient with a fulminating streptococcal infection. The patient was exceedingly contagious when Charles worked with him for about 15 minutes. The therapist had not been alerted to the potential danger and thus took no additional precautions to protect himself.

The infection was recognized by an ER physician. Charles had a fever of 103 degrees. His pulse was elevated. He looked terrible. The doctor didn't even need a stethoscope to appreciate her patient's respiratory congestion. Sputum was sent for culture and sensitivity studies. X-rays of the chest demonstrated cloudiness in multiple lobes of the lungs. Blood studies were sent off STAT, meaning get it done immediately. This was not any run-of-the-mill pneumonia. Charles was immediately admitted to John Muir Hospital in Walnut Creek, California.

Despite treatment with intravenous antibiotics, the lung infection was not responding as expected. In fact, the infection was not localized to just the lungs. Charles had contracted the "bug" through his respiratory system, but the bacteria were now circulating throughout his blood system. He had developed a septicemia. The infection had reached all of his extremities. A consulting infectious disease expert recommended transfer to a tertiary care facility, and UCSF Medical Center agreed to treat this acutely ill clinician. The hospital course was complicated after a determination was made that, to save his life, Charles would have to undergo multiple amputations. Both arms were removed just past the elbow. Both legs received below-the-knee amputations. The therapist was left with stumps after his wounds healed. He also underwent three plastic surgical procedures to his face where the infection had destroyed tissue. Not surprising, this man never again worked for pay.

Charles was recognized as having an industrial injury. The infection that almost killed him was caused by exposure to a hospital pathogen. The ER visit, the brief hospitalization at John Muir, the lengthy hospitalization at UCSF, the extensive physical therapy, the state-of-the-art prosthetics, and years of outpatient follow-up were all the responsibility of his employer and that hospital's insurer. Charles became a house husband and ran the family home while his wife continued her nursing career. He was Mr. Mom to his two kids. He adapted amazingly well. He didn't complain.

The purpose of my consult was to assist the insurer in determining whether the inpatient drug and alcohol rehabilitation that Charles had successfully completed should be considered the insurer's responsibility as well. He had never participated in mental health treatment before receiving care for his use of prescription opioids and alcohol. He showed no shame when shaking hands upon our meeting, me with my biologic hand and him with his titanium, electronic prosthesis. I learned quite a bit as a result of reviewing a dozen years of records and spending a couple of hours with Charles.

In complicated cases, I try to speak with the referral source, in addition to sending a written report addressing the areas of concern. In this case, the claims representative accepted my opinion that years of using pain medication and alcohol to deal with stump pain from four amputations had brought forth a state of chemical dependency. The substance abuse treatment costs were all due to the admitted exposure and infection.

What the insurance representative was not prepared for was my recommendation that Charles' upcoming cardiac surgery was also necessary care as a result of the industrial injury. The same bacteria that required amputations and reconstructive surgery had weakened a heart valve over time. To undergo the valve replacement procedure, a coronary bypass would also be necessary. I agreed that a cardiac specialist or infectious disease expert should be consulted rather than rely upon a psychiatrist, even one with a cell biology background. Needless to say, I have had no further referrals from that insurer. So, it goes, as the right thing was done for a truly injured worker. Once again, there is a reason psychiatrists go to medical school.

Charles' mind-set was key to understanding why he refused to play the victim. One can certainly imagine responding to his injury by becoming angry and resentful. Charles was neither. He was not preoccupied with the nursing staff neglecting to warn him of his patient's highly contagious state. He was not focused on the doctor who had ordered respiratory therapy without alerting staff to take special precautions. He showed no shame in his appearance despite having prosthetic devices on all four limbs. He was fully engaged in parental activities at his children's school. He remained involved in his community.

Rather than view himself as a recipient of past tragedy, Charles instead was active in the present. When asked how he maintained his demeanor, he commented that he had no choice but to be an example for his children in dealing with the cards one was dealt. He genuinely saw no other path but to stay involved. He had no place in his life for pity, anger, or despair. He had his bad days, especially when his amputation stump sites were sore, but he never felt either helpless or hopeless. He is a model of resilience.

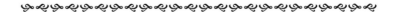

I first learned of Officer Young through the local news. He was a veteran police officer who had volunteered for duty on a multi-agency gang task force. In August 2010, Officer Young was in East Oakland, where he attempted to arrest a member of the Norteños gang on an outstanding warrant. A foot chase ensued. The suspect was armed. Gunshots were exchanged, and Officer Young was hit in the groin. A fellow officer tended to him until an ambulance arrived. Before accepting any analgesic medication, the wounded policeman gave details about his assailant, which went out on an all-points bulletin across the state. The officer was taken to a local trauma center where he was stabilized and underwent the first of many surgeries. He was later transferred to Stanford Hospital, where mesh was placed in his groin. Multiple hospitalizations took place, and his case was complicated by a persistent staphylococcus infection. Many months of physical therapy were necessary. Whereas his department expected Officer Young to retire, he began a vigorous course of strength and endurance training when his treating physician agreed it was safe to do so.

I reached out to Officer Young, whose story I found inspirational, and we developed a friendship over time. He initially presented as a well-developed, muscular guy with close-cropped hair. There was some concern about whether he would be fit psychologically to return to work in law enforcement, but nothing unusual came through in his answers to how he was doing emotionally. Of course, when we met, he carried a concealed weapon. Like other cops who worked in patrol, narcotics, SWAT, and gang unit assignments, there was no way this officer left home unarmed. He had seen too much violence during his career to leave himself vulnerable to bad guys.

Officer Young was also a "cop's cop" who never hesitated to respond to a critical incident, even when off duty. He reminded me of the officers who had jumped to my defense years ago when crazy, agitated patients in the ER tried to put me in the hospital. Officer Young had the mentality of a U.S. Marine. He went to war in urban settings where intravenous drug use, burglary, and prostitution were elements of the local economy. He was no choir boy, but most folks who knew him felt safe in his presence at a major sports event, rock concert, or other large public gathering.

Officer Young had managed to rehabilitate himself physically. He was left with chronic pain and numbness in his lower extremity and took medication to address the neurologic symptoms, but nothing that was habit forming. Psychologically, he mentioned minimal features of PTSD. He had had minimal contact with mental health providers during his hospitalizations. He had no interest in taking an antidepressant or going for counseling when the topic came up in our discussions. The information he provided just after having been shot led to the arrest of his assailant at the California-Mexico border. Officer Young testified at that gang member's trial, which resulted in a conviction for attempted murder of a police officer, punishable by a life sentence.

Officer Young wanted to resume his detective duties, and his department hoped he would be cleared to return. He was. Many months went by while he struggled with his pain, and his neurologic symptoms worsened due to his vigorous pursuit of police assignments. His treating physician, whom he trusted, told him he was increasing the chances that he would require further surgery and be left with greater limitations if he did not stop running after suspects and ending up in physical confrontations. Officer Young had one law enforcement setting, ALL IN. He retired in his late forties but remained an inspiration to younger officers who learned of his devotion to duty. Recently, he applied to a state university for training that would result in his becoming a high school PE teacher.

Officer Young displayed characteristics of hardiness wherein the theme of "mind over matter" played out. No one would ask to be shot and almost die. Like Charles, Officer Young played the cards he was dealt. He did so for his fellow officers, his family, and himself. He never described being moody, belligerent, or rude while repeatedly being subjected to uncomfortable procedures. At no point did he consider himself a victim, though statistically he was labeled as such. When he retired from law enforcement, it was with reluctance, but not shame. He was proud of having been of service. He never regretted his decision to become a cop.

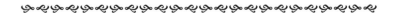

    I believe most of us would prefer to be seen as survivors rather than victims when life-threatening events come our way. Basic biology and genetic predisposition are factors in how we react to such occurrences. My mother would tell me that how we're raised matters too. Training and life experience can help prepare us to respond as selfless or selfish. Similarly, how our society treats those involved in critical incidents or catastrophes must also influence how fellow citizens respond. How would you fare on the "impaired victim to courageous survivor" continuum, should unexpected tragedy come your way?

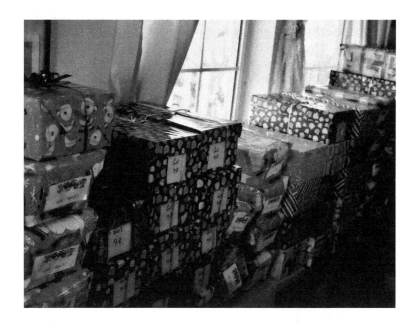

36 | Giving Back

> ❝ **At the end of the day it's not about what you have or even what you've accomplished. ...It's about who you've lifted up, who you've made better. It's about what you've given back.**❞
> *— Denzel Washington*

It's never too late to give back. Little acts of kindness inspire generosity. It's contagious. Theon Johnson III, a friend of mine, is a Methodist minister who recently gave a sermon on giving back. He said, "A mind-set of scarcity is a barrier to a life of generosity." How will you be judged? Will your acts show you to have paid back some of what you've been fortunate enough to have received? When considering the importance of work in our lives, is there room for giving to others through our labor? Does our job provide sufficiently that we can share with those in our community? A full, balanced life is measured by what we produce yet also by what we relinquish.

"Unless someone like you cares a whole awful lot, nothing is going to get better. It's not."
— Dr. Seuss

Throughout my career as a psychiatrist for working people who have suffered physical injury and emotional trauma on the job, I have been blessed. The challenges these fellow citizens have confronted often have been daunting. My job is to assist those in need to receive the care they are due. It is also to encourage them to not give up, to persevere. If I do my job as observer and coach, then these brothers and sisters might see opportunity where they previously saw no future.

"Not only must we be good, but we must be good for something."
— Henry David Thoreau

Growing up in the Chicago area, we were often introduced to adults by learning what kind of work they did. There was no shame in having a job that emphasized physical strength. Being a general manager might have paid well, but everyone understood what a carpenter or a trucker did. Being good for something tangible is highly valuable.

"We make a living by what we get, but we make a life by what we give."
— Winston Churchill

Being a health care provider is filled with intimate contacts with folks desperate for help and understanding. Yet as a physician, obligations can interfere with being present with a patient. The requirements for documentation, knowing and abiding by the rules of a modern healthcare system, keeping up with clinical advances, and the reality of getting reimbursed can cause doctors to lose perspective. It can also become a game about publishing manuscripts, giving lectures, and reaping financial rewards. Giving to those in need can become secondary.

"It's easy to make a buck. It's a lot tougher to make a difference."
— Tom Brokaw

Over my four decades in medicine, I have seen doctors who have made a difference in the lives of others. These individuals might or might not be distinguished professors. They might or might not live in the best part of town. To make a difference they have invariably cared deeply for those who trust their lives to them. A physician who makes a difference, remains mindful of the promise, and oath, to do no harm. If an error occurs, own it and fix it, if one can. I recall the chairman of my department counseling me and my fellow residents: "Patients will forgive us for mistakes of the mind, but not the heart." A doctor who truly cares about a patient's outcome does not do so as a reflection of ego, but as an expression of mutual respect. In that scenario, I am my brother's keeper.

"Even if it's a little thing, do something for those who have need of a man's help — something for which you get no pay but the privilege of doing it. For, remember you don't live in a world all your own. Your brothers are here too."
— *Albert Schweitzer*

At times, I have considered how different life might have been had I taken another path. I could have pursued additional training in science rather than go to medical school. I might have dropped out of college to become a partner in a start-up company that is now a multi-billion-dollar food producer. I could have taken a paid faculty position like peers I knew. In the end, we are not defined by the particular product or service we create, but rather by the manner in which we affect those we serve. If you are engaging in meaningful work, those for whom you provide service will decide your value.

"The best way to find yourself is to lose yourself in the service of others."
— *Mahatma Gandhi*

When our office is doing things correctly, we are part of a system that helps injured workers to once again become productive. At times, this is through recommending treatment that allows for healing and for a return to the worker's normal duties, since most employees with emotional problems can benefit from time-limited counseling and being reunited with their work group. A return to productivity can also result from recommending practical accommodations an employer can implement. By way of example, an iron worker developed acrophobia, a fear of heights, following a fall at a construction site. After his physical injuries healed, he returned to work, through assistance from his union, at jobs that were at ground level. Many workers who remain impaired for normal duty come to see value in another career path. A retail clerk who has been the victim of an armed robbery can avoid the possibility of a recurrence by taking a job that requires no money handling. At our offices, we help workers get back to being functional.

"As you grow older, you will discover that you have two hands — one for helping yourself, the other for helping others."
— *Audrey Hepburn*

When a worker cannot go back to work, life is not over even though it can feel that way. The disabled are still capable of providing service. Retirees don't need to wait around for death to come knocking at their door. Volunteering is available. Many non-profit agencies rely upon volunteers to stock shelves in food banks, give docent tours at museums, make home visits to the housebound, and coach youth athletics. The fact there might not be a paycheck does not diminish the work done. Yes, it is work, God's work.

> **"I've learned that you shouldn't go through life with a catcher's mitt on both hands. You need to be able to throw something back."**
> — *Maya Angelou*

Well-being is in part the result of acts of selflessness. When heroes are recognized for putting the lives of others above their own interests, we are inspired. Should we be so fortunate to be the subject of a police officer's or a firefighter's courage, then we have an obligation to do more than say, "Thank you." Through action we pay back what grace has come our way. When I became president of the California Society of Industrial Medicine and Surgery, a state occupational medicine association, all members in attendance were asked to again take the Hippocratic oath. The point was to remind colleagues that duties come with the privilege of caring for the health of others. We should give thanks to our patients for entrusting their precious lives unto our skills and acumen.

> **"Life's most persistent and urgent question is, what are you doing for others?"**
> — *Martin Luther King, Jr.*

Thankfully, the career of a physician allows one to give back over and over, provided the work is taken seriously. Doctors are competitive professionals. They often have big egos. When at their best, their complete focus is on the person they are listening to and touching during the examination, and for whom they are providing advocacy. In occupational psychiatry, our patients run a gamut from having no prior contact with a mental health practitioner to having had years of psychotherapy. Our patients are immigrants and Americans whose relatives fought in our Civil War. Some are illiterate, while others have advanced degrees. To be a successful occupational psychiatrist, one must find common ground with the individual who seeks relief from emotional distress. Walk a mile in that brother's moccasins.

> **"The meaning of life is to find yourself. The purpose to life is to give it away."**
> — *William Shakespeare*

A path was taken. Numerous stories were told. A kid from Chicago grew up and explored the world. He took in information like a sponge. He saw how working people developed pride in producing goods and services, and he saw how they could fall upon misfortune by just doing their jobs. He had the opportunity to make recommendations about career options. At times, he assisted some to transition in their work life and to find a place for memories, both good and bad, to have a home.

> **"Service to others is the rent you pay for your room here on Earth."**
> — *Muhammad Ali*

ACKNOWLEDGMENTS

My career has been spent as a physician and psychiatrist serving an employee population that has paid a high price for doing their jobs. These tales speak for themselves and hopefully convince those who read them to recognize the sacrifices made.

To my wife Kim, I owe much for encouraging me through the writing project which resulted in *Wounded Workers*. She helped immeasurably in her recommendations of which sagas to depict and in her multiple edits and reviews of the manuscript. My office manager, Wendy Lemberg, proofed and formatted early versions of the book. She kept the cases organized and secure while assisting with gathering information and facilitating my collaboration with project partners.

A number of colleagues have reviewed and critiqued elements of the manuscript. Dr. Steve Sharfstein was enthusiastic about the book's value, while Dr. Don Fidler a psychiatrist and playwright, emphasized the need to end up with a quality product as a positive reflection on the topic of the American worker. Dr. Victor Reus was spot on with his remarks that led to an improved book and the recognition that my views might not be universally shared by other psychiatrists. My longtime friend Dr. Gary Wise was kind in his review while reminding me of the facts underlying the science portrayed in the book.

After arriving upon a title, there was also a need to design the book's cover. Gifted artist Pedro Silva assisted with its early versions. It was the sincere efforts of Bill Thompson of the Thompson Marketing Group that resulted in the final cover design and the launching of my website.

Finally, it was only through the efforts of my publishing consultant, Karen Bomm, that a raw manuscript was transformed into a published book. Jeff Braucher helped to clean up the submission for printing through his assistance with proofreading. Kathy Haq steered the project in the right direction with her journalistic advice. Jody Hucko has proven invaluable in getting punctuation and sentence structure better. Additional proofreading was provided by a colleague Marisa Huston.

Yet another colleague, Dr. Bill Reid, strongly recommended the services of a professional editor after his preliminary review of an advanced reader copy of the book. That led to my friend and best-selling author, Anne Hillerman, referring me to Daddy Wags Editing. It is as the result of Jim Wagner's meticulous edits that the content flows along. Only through the skillful formatting performed by Dree Morin of Dreemer Designs was the manuscript enabled for print and ebook publication. It takes a team effort to build a book. My team and I hope that *Wounded Workers* is favorably received by you, an audience of workers and clinicians alike.

With gratitude for making true tales come to life.

Dr. Bob Larsen

ABOUT THE AUTHOR

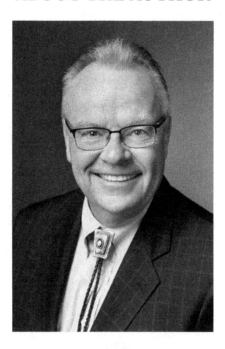

Over a career of four decades, Dr. Bob Larsen has evaluated, treated, and advocated for multitudes of injured workers. After presenting to audiences of clinicians and the general public, and publishing in professional journals and textbooks, Dr. Bob completed his first book project, a compendium of cases of employees challenged by real-life disasters played out in the workplace. Dr. Bob speaks through vignettes of workers confronted with a myriad of employment incidents, causing us to consider the subjects of job stress, PTSD, emotional resilience, delayed recovery, harassment, workplace violence, and much more.

Dr. Bob grew up a working-class kid in the Chicago area. He headed west to train as a cell biologist at the University of Colorado. He later engaged in basic science research at the University of Miami and at Boston University. He went on to teach microbiology to his classmates at Northwestern University Medical School. While in medical school, Dr. Bob first explored the fields of psychiatry and psychology. He was drawn to working in mental health because it required an understanding of biology and medicine while addressing complex disturbances of emotion, behavior, perception, thoughts, and interpersonal relationships.

Following residency training at the University of California, San Francisco (UCSF), a fellowship in health policy at UCSF/Stanford, and graduate studies in healthcare administration at the University of California at Berkeley, Dr. Bob opted to take a hands-on approach to workers injured while doing their jobs. These workers have come to his offices from manufacturing, the service sector, management, law enforcement, farming, and high-tech industries. Their reasons are never pretty: robberies, shootings, amputations, burn injuries, motor vehicle accidents, and other horrors too numerous to mention. His job is to develop a plan for dealing with the flashbacks, guilt, insecurity, fears, and damaged self-image that follow these real tragedies.

Dr. Bob has been a treating physician, a health policy advocate, an educator, and a forensic psychiatrist. He is a clinical professor of psychiatry at UCSF. He founded the Center for Occupational Psychiatry in 1985 and is a past president of the California Society of Industrial Medicine and Surgery. His body of professional work is now portrayed in *Wounded Workers*, which brings to life the sacrifices American workers make in doing their jobs, jobs that are frequently more dangerous than commonly known or acknowledged.

Aside from his clinical work, writing, and speaking engagements as a psychiatrist and professor, Dr. Bob enjoys sharing life experiences with his wife Kim in the community of Santa Fe, New Mexico. As a balance to the inevitable burden associated with assisting others in dealing with work-related tragedy, his interests in photography, travel, blues music, and baseball allow Dr. Bob to "keep on keepin' on." Travel, baseball, and music have become far more limited since COVID-19 arrived. Photography, biking, and gardening have had to suffice.

For additional information on Dr. Bob Larsen, visit his website at http://workingmansshrink.com.

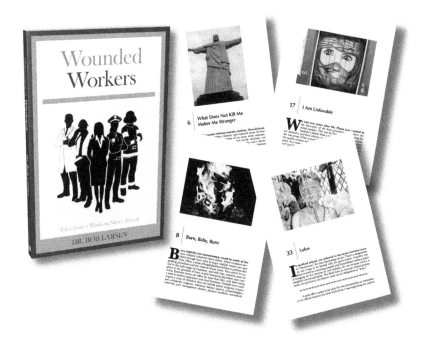

Additional thoughts:

Now that you've finished reading Wounded Workers, you may, no doubt, feel a range of emotions. The plight, courage, and persistence of these victims range from heartbreaking to inspirational.

You might know someone, a neighbor, friend, family member or coworker who can relate to any one of these tales. If you do, please let them know they are not alone. I will share ways you can continue to keep in touch, connect with me as I write my Musings, and provide updates on future publications and appearances.

WorkingMansShrink.com

CPSIA information can be obtained
at www.ICGtesting.com
Printed in the USA
BVHW092254150822
644633BV00002B/11